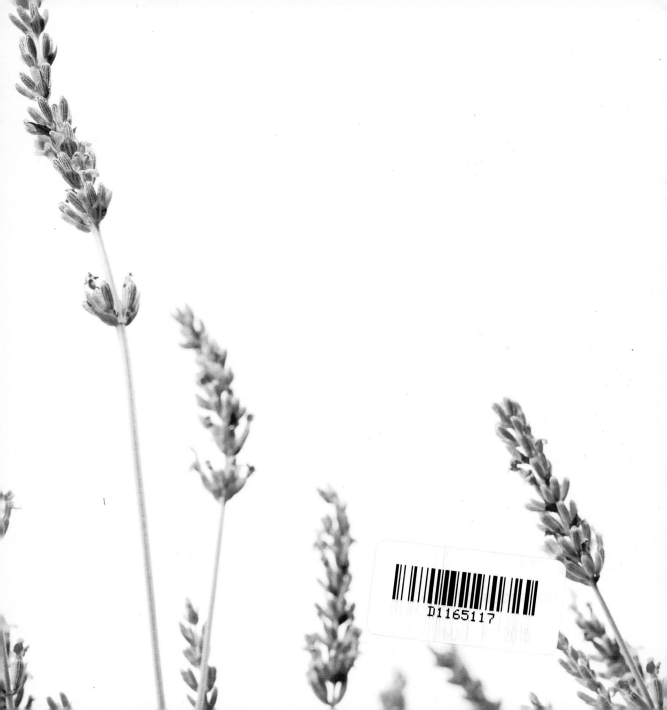

D1165117

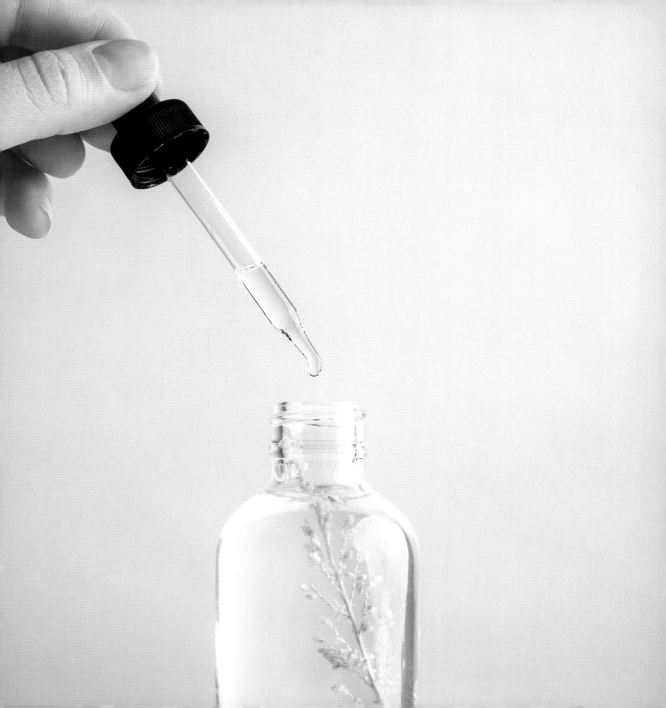

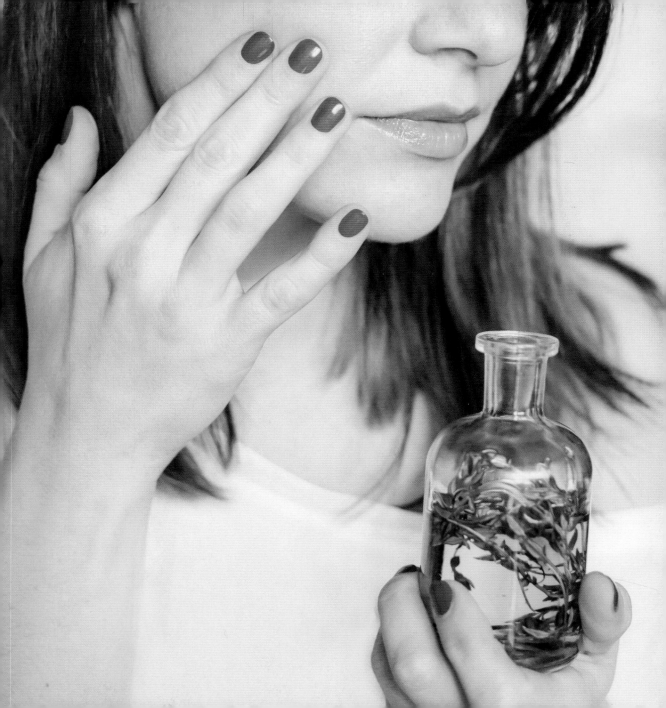

ESSENTIAL
glow

Stephanie Gerber
of Hello Glow

weldon**owen**

Contents

Soothe

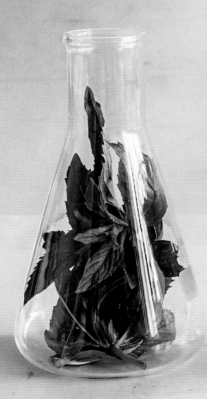
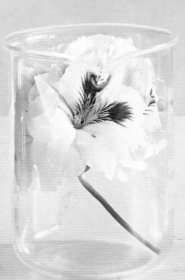
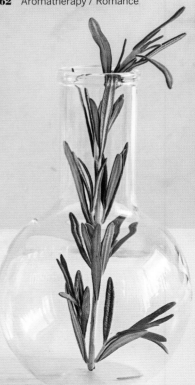

Introduction

Like a lot of people, lavender was my first essential oil. It seemed like a good place to start—it smells amazing and has a million uses, give or take a few! Next I tried peppermint and eucalyptus, then lemon and tea tree, and now I'm a little afraid to know how many essential oils are in my collection. But those first five created a solid foundation for tons of first-aid recipes, skincare concoctions, and homemade green-cleaning formulas.

Before I started learning about essential oils' therapeutic uses, I was drawn to their pleasing aromas. The exotic scents of ylang ylang and jasmine. The clean, woodsy notes of juniper and pine, which make me think of long walks in the crisp fall air. The bright, uplifting fragrances of grapefruit, lime, and sweet orange. Your sense of smell is powerful, so start by using your own nose to select the essential oils that improve your mood—that make you feel fresh, delicate, sexy, you name it!

But know that the applications for essential oils go so much farther than mere perfume. Using these distillations in a holistic program for your body and spirit is at the heart of aromatherapy, and this book is designed to help you incorporate these helpful elixirs into your daily life. I've broken down the benefits of more than 20 of the most popular

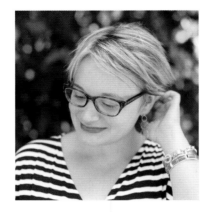

essential oils, and for each offered easy, effective recipes for wellness, beauty, and home that help you get the most of their individual powers and properties. (Psst: Many recipes call for a few essential oils—so you'll get to explore more than 40 total—but the featured oil is always the most prominent in the blend.)

The active compounds in essential oils can help majorly expand your wellness repertoire—from helping your body heal minor scrapes and cuts to kicking a headache, acne, or PMS. They'll also help you create a cooling spray to relieve sunburn, give yourself a massage to ease achy muscles after a workout, or apply a hydrating mask to dull and dry skin.

As you explore essential oils, aromatherapy will become a key part of the self-care rituals that contribute

to your overall health. You can support your sleep by spritzing a calming room spray or drawing an aromatic bath. Craft DIY cleaners to reduce the toxin load in your home, or enhance a stress-reducing meditation or yoga practice with grounding essential oils.

I've also covered the basic usage guidelines—these oils can be potent, so selecting, diluting, and storing them properly is crucial to a safe and positive experience. Plus, some aren't recommended for people of certain ages or with specific medical concerns; to reap the benefits, you've got to heed this advice!

But there's also plenty of fun advice in this book's pages. You'll soon find yourself playing mixologist, concocting new favorite fragrances and blends that target all kinds of everyday wants and desires (from making your home smell zesty fresh to freshening up your love life). There's also a quick-look guide to selecting the best essential oils for life's minor trials and tribulations.

Clean living and conscientious beauty rituals mean caring about the ingredients you use in your house and on your skin. My goal is to give you practical, enjoyable ways to care for yourself, your family, and your home. And, of course, to make everything smell absolutely amazing!

Stephanie Gruber

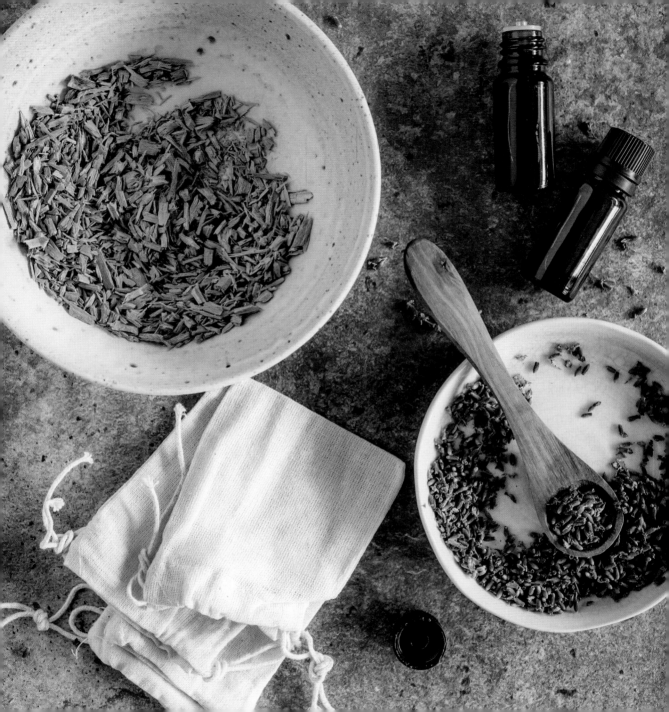

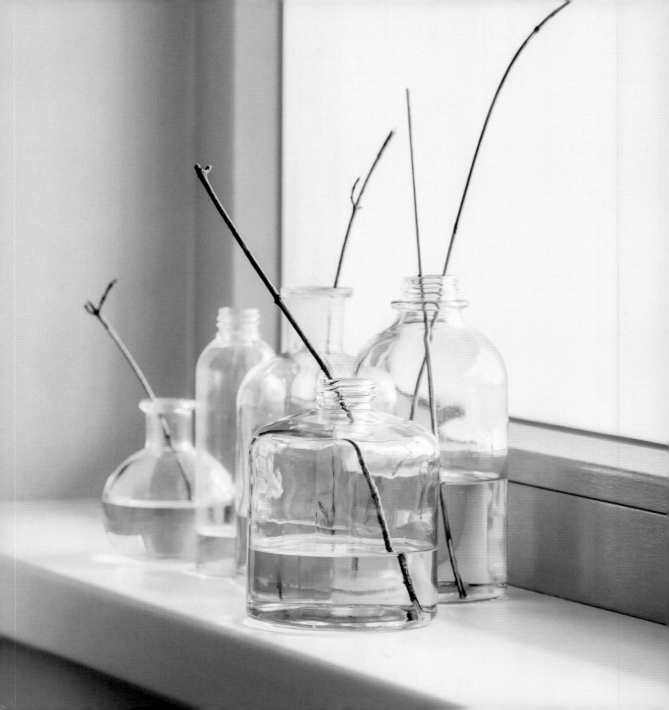

Essential Oils 101

The popularity of essential oils has skyrocketed in recent years as people have increasingly looked for natural ways to take control of their well-being. But these helpful elixirs can be overwhelming—with so many to choose from, which ones do you really need? Take a deep breath: I'm going to explain what these powerful oils are all about, as well as how to select, use, and store them.

What are essential oils?

An essential oil is a highly concentrated plant extract that contains active chemical compounds, the most common of which are hydrocarbons in the form of terpenes. These compounds team up to give a plant a particular aroma, which plants produce to attract pollinators, defend against insects or other plants, or protect from bacterial or fungal attacks. These chemical agents also lend essential oils their antiseptic, anti-inflammatory, and antiviral properties—that's right, they do more than just smell good!

Unlike cooking oils, essential oils feel light and nongreasy. They're also highly volatile, meaning that they quickly turn to vapor and evaporate when heated. They dissolve in other oils, alcohols, honey, and milk (but not in water).

Essential oils may be extracted from flowers, leaves, seeds, or berries. Rose essential oil, for example, comes from petals (it takes 1,000 to make one tiny bottle!), while citrus essential oils are drawn from the peel and eucalyptus essential oil originates in the leaf. The most common method of extracting this so-called essence is distillation, the process by which plants inside a high-pressure still are subjected to steam or water, which softens the organic matter so that the oils can be extracted and separated from the water. Another common process is cold-press, or expression: The organic matter undergoes extreme pressure and rotation, which batters it and makes it release oil. Oils from fragile plants like jasmine, gardenia, rose, and neroli are sometimes extracted using a solvent, which creates an absolute.

What are their benefits?

"The way to health is to have an aromatic bath and scented massage every day," said Hippocrates, the Greek physician considered the founding father of natural medicine. And, 2,500 years later, who can argue with that?

Essential oils generally work in two ways. First, they have powerful aromas. When we inhale one of their scents, it sends messages to our brains' olfactory bulbs, affecting emotions and the limbic system (the part of the brain that controls memory), as well as breathing, blood circulation, and hormones. Second, essential oils' small molecular structures allow them to penetrate the skin more easily than other vegetable or nut oils, which stay on the skin's surface; this trait makes essential oils ideal for topical application. The tiny molecules work their way into the bloodstream and lymphatic system, treating aches and pains or repairing scars and skin tissue. (Essential oils are too concentrated to be applied directly to the skin, however, and must be diluted in a carrier oil or liquid; see page 11 for more information.)

How do you use essential oils?

Essential oils are helpful in a myriad of applications. Here are a few common ways to add them to your daily routine.

DIFFUSION A reed diffuser, room spray, or steam vaporizer allows you to fill your environment with the aromas of essential oils. You can buy a diffuser—several stylish models are readily available from major retailers and online—or fashion your own (see page 30).

INHALATION There are several ways to breathe in the benefits! Apply 1 or 2 drops to a handkerchief, carry it in your pocket, and pull it out to inhale the aroma, reviving your energy or resetting your mood whenever you like. You can also sprinkle a few drops on your pillow at night. For an effective steam treatment, add 1 or 2 drops to a bowl filled with 3 cups (710 mL) boiling water. Place a towel over your head and the bowl, and breathe deeply for no more than 10 minutes. (Get the OK from your doctor before using any essential oil if you have asthma or other respiratory issues.)

BATH Dilute 4 to 6 drops essential oil in 1 teaspoon carrier oil, milk, honey, or unscented liquid castile soap, and add to a warm bath. You'll get the aromatherapy benefits while absorbing the essential oils through your skin. Some essential oils—like cinnamon leaf, clove bud, ginger, and oregano—can irritate sensitive skin, so increase the dilution or avoid using these oils topically.

MASSAGE For a relaxing at-home massage oil, add 4 to 6 drops essential oil to 2 teaspoons carrier oil (such as grape-seed or sweet almond). Start with a scalp massage if you want the oils to quickly enter the bloodstream, then move onto the shoulders, back, feet, and more.

COMPRESS A cool compress is always a soothing treat for irritated skin—whether it's puffy eyes or a sunburn. Add 2 or 3 drops of an anti-inflammatory essential oil (like Roman chamomile) to 3 cups (710 mL) water. Soak a washcloth in the mixture, wring it out, and apply to the affected area.

Selecting essential oils

When starting your collection, don't buy a dozen at once—you'll find them unused months later (like I did). Instead, start with one or two classics (like tea tree, lavender, or lemon) that have a wide range of uses for wellness, home, and beauty. Then add one or two more oils at a time as you discover your favorites.

When it comes to quality, look for essential oils that are naturally derived via distillation or expression and that come with no added ingredients. If there's an alcohol or a preservative listed on the label, steer clear. There are many synthetic and low-quality oils on the market, so do your research and buy direct from distillers or well-trusted brands.

It's crucial to purchase only oils that say "100 percent pure" on the label. Pure oils seem expensive, but you'll only use a few drops per recipe, so a small bottle will last a long time. If a pricey pure oil (like rose or jasmine) is out of your budget, look for it prediluted in a carrier oil or its main ingredient in a blend of other essential oils.

Keep in mind that fragrance and perfume oils are not the same as essential oils. They have no therapeutic benefits. Skip these!

Storing essential oils

Light, heat, moisture, and oxygen can harm essential oils, so store yours in blue or amber glass bottles, and keep them in a cool, dark spot. Don't use plastic containers, as both the bottle and the oil will degrade. Keeping the bottles tightly closed and replacing the caps quickly after use will also help prevent evaporation and oxidation.

In general, essential oils will keep for at least 1 year. Citrus oils will start to lose their powers after 2 years, but floral, herbal, and wood oils can last 4 or more. When mixed with carrier oils, however, your concoctions will have a shorter shelf life, so make them in small batches and use them within 6 months (or as specified in your recipe). Always label your blends with the recipe ingredients and expiration dates.

When making beauty treatments using essential oils, be sure you sterilize all glass containers before storing your recipes in them. Wash them in hot soapy water or boil them for 20 minutes, then dry thoroughly.

A Few Words on Safety

Essential oils are very concentrated, so it's important to follow all safety guidelines on the labels and consult with your physician when adding them to your wellness routine. Here are some best practices.

Always dilute

To avoid irritation, you should never apply essential oils directly to your skin without first diluting them with a carrier oil, such as sweet almond or grape-seed (see page 18 for more about carrier oils). These base oils trap the essential oils, inhibiting their evaporation, and allow them to be absorbed through the pores. In general, you should always stick with a low dilution of 1 to 3 percent. A 1 percent dilution rate—1 drop essential oil per 1 teaspoon carrier oil—is recommended for daily face applications, children over age 6, pregnant women, elderly adults, and those who have sensitive or damaged skin. (These folks should also start with essential oils that rarely cause irritation, like Roman chamomile, lavender, patchouli, and frankincense.) Healthy adults with healthy skin can use a 2 percent dilution rate—2 drops per 1 teaspoon essential oil—in most topical treatments, like massage oils and body lotions. Higher dilutions come in to play for localized conditions like muscle aches.

(One exception: Lavender is considered safe to apply to the skin "neat"—aka, without dilution—but check with your doctor first.)

Never ingest

Essential oils aren't appropriate to drink or eat, unless your doctor advises it. If you've incorporated an essential oil into a DIY mouthwash or throat gargle, be sure to dilute it (2 drops per 1 cup/240 mL water) and always spit it all out.

Keep away from kids

Do not use essential oils on children under 2 years old; a dilution of 0.25 percent (that's 1 drop essential oil per 4 teaspoons carrier oil) is recommended up to age 6. After age 6, a 1 percent dilution is fine. Some essential oils (such as eucalyptus and rosemary) are not safe for kids, so consult with your pediatrician first. Lock your essential oils in a cabinet away from little hands.

Start with a patch test

It's wise to do a patch test with all essential oils before including them in a topical treatment, and that goes double if an oil is known to irritate dry or sensitive skin. Some essential oils—like cinnamon leaf, clove bud, and oregano—can cause redness or blotchiness, so avoid using these on inflamed or damaged skin. Likewise,

refrain from applying peppermint, cinnamon leaf, or lemongrass near the mouth, eyes, or nose, as these essential oils tend to irritate mucous membranes. To conduct a patch test before use, dilute 1 drop essential oil with 1 teaspoon carrier oil and apply to an inconspicuous spot, such as your chest or inner arm. If there's no skin reaction after 24 hours, the essential oil should be fine to use.

Consult if pregnant

Many essential oils are not recommended for use if you're nursing or during pregnancy, especially in the early months. Check with your doctor before use.

Avoid your eyes

Take care to avoid getting essential oils in your peepers. Flush them out right away with water if you do.

Avoid the sun

Some citrus essential oils are phototoxic, meaning they can make your skin susceptible to sunburn. If you've applied one, avoid spending time in the sun for at least 12 hours.

Watch for allergies

Use of an essential oil over time can result in an allergic reaction. If you think you've become sensitized to an essential oil, isolate it in a patch test in an inconspicuous spot.

The Art of Aromatherapy

When paired correctly, multiple essential oils can team up to create pleasing aromas and more effective treatments. If you're just starting to play mixologist, follow this general road map to aromatic bliss.

Home in on a problem

Many popular essential oil blends are formulated for specific issues, like staving off a chest cold or clearing up acne. Others are all about providing emotional support through the power of scent. If you hope to combat either a physical or an emotional problem with your blend, do your research to see which essential oils will do the trick. (See pages 176–179 for a list of common ailments and their essential oil fixes.) Select one that works with your primary goal to act as the foundation of your aromatherapy blend. (If you're just looking for a lovely signature scent, you can skip the research and simply choose an essential oil that appeals to you.)

Add oils to enhance your blend

Whether you're looking to solve a problem or just smell a bit nicer, see the chart on pages 14–15 to determine the categories of your potential oils; this will help you make some decisions about which might mingle nicely. In general,
essential oils from the same categories tend to play well with one another (citrus with citrus, floral with floral, and so on), while other pairs should complement or contrast. For example, citrus and herbaceous oils tend to harmonize, while spicy and floral ones tend to set each other off. You can also add essential oils that will enhance the wellness goal of your blend. If you're using, say, lavender to relieve stress, blend it with other soothing oils, such as Roman chamomile or clary sage.

Play with mixes

It's best to keep your blends to three to five essential oils at first. An easy way to test a combination's scent is by waving the bottles under your nose. If you don't like the scent, just try a different pairing. Another consideration is how long certain scents will last. Essential oils are often classified into three categories according to how long they take to evaporate. Top notes tend to perk up your nose right away, but their small molecules evaporate within minutes. Middle notes add staying power and richness to a blend, while base notes tend to be strong aromatics that calm and relax—their scents last the longest. Ideally, your scent will include all three notes, but don't limit yourself! (See page 89 for a list of top, middle, and bottom notes.)

Perfect your ratios

Once you've fallen for a combo, tinker with the exact measurements to get the formula just so. Here, the philosophies really differ. Some find it useful to start with equal percentages of each essential oil and adjust from there based on their potency (watch out, because strong oils will overpower the whole blend!). For fragrance blending, the rule of thumb is to use a ratio of 30 percent top note, 50 percent middle note, and 20 percent base note. Whichever route you take, blend the oils together in a glass bottle and note how the scent changes over 48 hours. Don't forget to label your creation with the ingredients and measurements so you can easily re-create the mix.

Decide on a delivery method

Finally, think about how you want to use your essential oil blend. You can diffuse your blend and breathe in its benefits; use it in a household cleaner or decorative craft; or deliver it topically in a massage oil, a creamy salve, or an aromatic bath. If you intend to use your creation directly on your skin, be sure to follow the dilution guidelines on page 11 and talk to your doctor or aromatherapist before use.

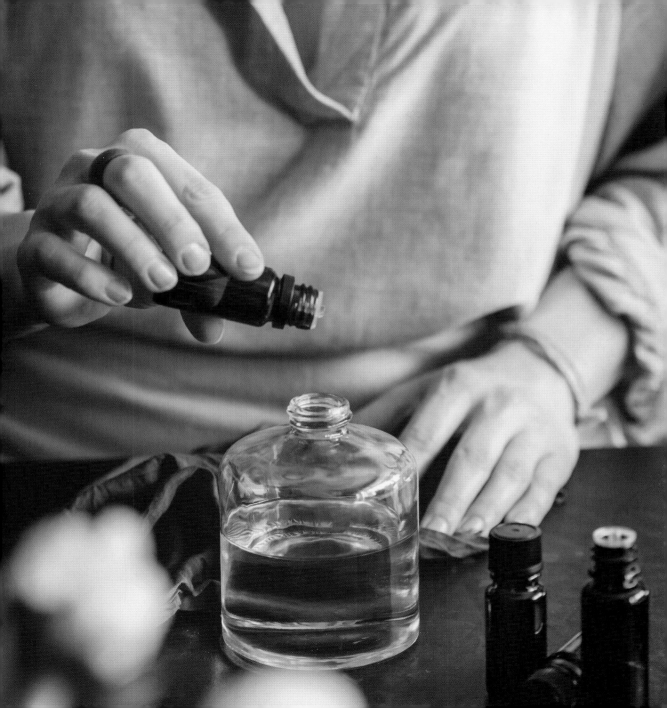

Know Your Scent Categories

Before mixing up a blend, pause to consider these aroma types. Using essential oils from the same group in your blend can create an agreeable, harmonizing mix, or you can try playing different categories off each other for more complex aromas. (You'll also want to play around with top, middle, and bottom notes; see page 89 for a breakdown of where common essential oils fall in this classification.) As you experiment, keep a journal to track your ratios—and your reactions to them—so you'll be able to replicate your new favorite scents. If you feel overwhelmed, look at the label on a blend you really love and see what you can learn from its ingredients list.

CITRUS

Bright, cheerful scents energize and perk you up.

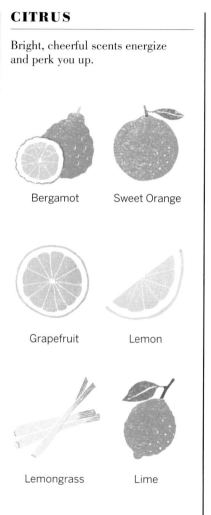

Bergamot   Sweet Orange

Grapefruit   Lemon

Lemongrass   Lime

FLORAL

These sweet floral essential oils are classic scents in feminine perfumes.

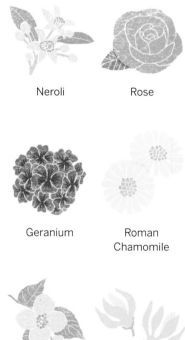

Neroli   Rose

Geranium   Roman Chamomile

Jasmine   Ylang Ylang

HERBAL

Fresh menthol aromas invigorate and improve focus.

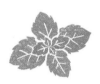

Peppermint

Rosemary

Eucalyptus

Sweet Basil

Tea Tree

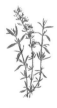

Hyssop

SPICY

A little goes a long way with these spicy, sensual, and warming aromas.

Cinnamon Leaf

Clove Bud

Clary Sage

Thyme

Ginger

Black Pepper

WOODSY

These earthy scents are strengthening and balancing, and they often skew masculine.

Cedarwood

Sandalwood

Frankincense

Juniper

Pine

Vetiver

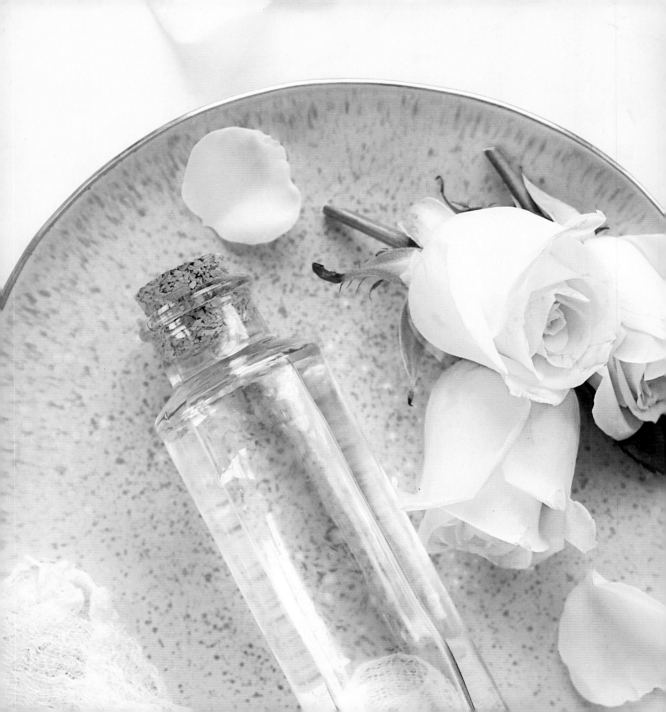

Making Your Own Oils

Homemade Infused Oils

½ cup (20 g) dried herbs, such as arnica, calendula, chamomile, comfrey, green tea, or lavender

1 cup (240 mL) carrier oil, such as coconut, grape-seed, or sweet almond

8-ounce (240-mL) jar

My do-it-yourself attempts at distilling essential oils have all ended in tears, mold, and wasted herbs, so I recommend making infused oils instead. While not as potent, these carrier oils are fantastic in healing balms, lotions, and salves.

STEP 1 / Pour 2 inches (5 cm) of water into a saucepan and bring it to a boil. Reduce the heat to low.

STEP 2 / Mix the herbs and oil in a heat-safe glass bowl. Place it over the saucepan and simmer for 1 hour, stirring often. Avoid overheating, which can reduce the benefits. Add water to the saucepan as needed.

STEP 3 / Remove the mixture from heat and let it cool. Filter it with a fine-mesh strainer, squeezing out as much oil as you can. Discard the herbs.

STEP 4 / Transfer the oil to a jar. If strained properly, it should last up to 2 years.

DIY Aromatic Hydrosol

2 cups (60 g) fresh flower petals, herbs, or fruit peels

4 cups (945 mL) distilled water

Ice

Capture the fragrance of beloved herbs, flowers, or fruit peels in a hydrosol—a floral or herbal water that lends a lovely scent and organic compounds to all-natural recipes. Try rose petals in a skin toner, lemon peels and thyme in a cleaning spray, or lavender flowers in a pillow mist to encourage sleep.

STEP 1 / Arrange a heat-safe glass bowl in the center of a large stock pot. Place your petals, herbs, or peels around the bowl, then pour the distilled water over the botanicals.

STEP 2 / Using a domed lid with a handle, cover the pot so that the lid is upside-down. Center a large chunk of ice on top of the lid.

STEP 3 / Bring the water to a simmer, letting the condensation that forms on the lid's underside drip into the small bowl inside the pot for 25 to 30 minutes. Replace the ice as it melts.

STEP 4 / Remove the bowl—which will now be filled with your herbal water—and let it cool before use.

Stocking an All-Natural Pantry

Complement your essential oil kit with these organic ingredients and basic kitchen tools.

Carrier oils

These unrefined plant-based extracts from nuts or seeds play a crucial role in diluting their essential cousins, but they're also great ingredients in their own right.

COCONUT A great carrier oil for most skin types is coconut oil. Rich in vitamin E, antioxidants, and fatty acids, it hydrates dry skin and can help reduce the appearance of cellulite, stretch marks, and rough skin patches.

GRAPE-SEED An excellent regulator of the body's oil production, grape-seed oil is full of antioxidants and vitamin C, making it great at fighting adult acne. It also helps restore collagen and calms skin inflammation.

JOJOBA Made from jojoba seeds, this popular oil works for all skin types. Full of fatty acids and vitamin E, it moisturizes without leaving a heavy residue.

SWEET ALMOND This gentle, lightly scented oil is rich in vitamin E, fatty acids, proteins, and minerals. It's an extra-moisturizing treat for very dry or sensitive skin.

Other natural ingredients

You'll find most of these in your kitchen or bathroom cabinets. Buy organic versions, if possible.

VINEGAR Antibacterial and antiseptic, both apple cider and distilled white vinegar are fantastic disinfectants. ACV is chock-full of natural alpha hydroxy acids, which help exfoliate dead skin cells, while distilled white vinegar is a cheap go-to ingredient in green cleaners.

ALOE VERA When taken straight from the plant, soothing and cooling aloe vera gel contains high levels of amino acids, minerals, and vitamins.

BAKING SODA This cheap stuff absorbs anything, making it a fantastic ingredient in cleansers—for your face or your tub! Baking soda can also ease skin irritation.

BEESWAX Often used to thicken balms, this natural bee product seals in moisture. Plus, it has antibacterial and antifungal properties.

CASTILE Use this plant-derived, biodegradable soap in body washes and household cleaners alike.

CLAY Known for its ability to draw out toxins, clay also tightens and tones skin. Many can jump-start circulation to reduce puffiness.

COCOA BUTTER This delicious-smelling moisturizer coats the skin. Its vitamin E can improve skin tone and help prevent stretch marks.

EPSOM SALT This wonder-worker can soothe muscle pain and aches, relieve the itch of sunburn and poison ivy, decrease swelling, and boost your body's magnesium levels.

HONEY This sweet stuff is antibacterial, antifungal, and antiseptic. It helps your skin retain moisture—and glow!

LEMON Citrus juice is an effective astringent—plus it can kick-start your body's lymphatic system. It also makes a fantastic natural cleaner.

SHEA BUTTER Softer than cocoa butter, shea has a silky texture that's easily absorbed by the skin. Its vitamins A and E restore elasticity.

Simple tools

Dedicate a set of tools for your essential oil experiments. Before use, clean them with isopropyl alcohol to prevent bacterial contamination.
- Measuring cups and spoons
- Nesting heat-safe glass bowls
- Double boiler (or a saucepan and a heat-safe bowl that fits inside)
- Pipette or eyedropper
- Fine-mesh strainer or cheesecloth
- Blue or amber 5-mL glass bottles

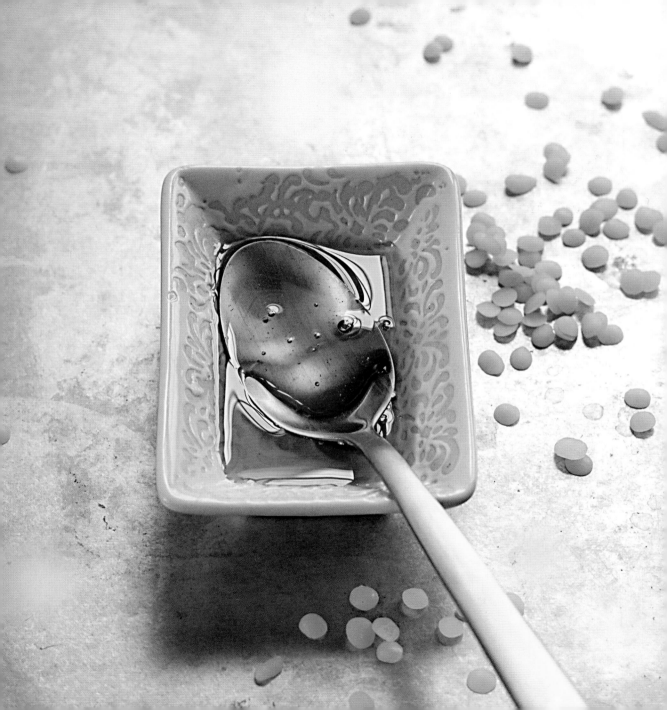

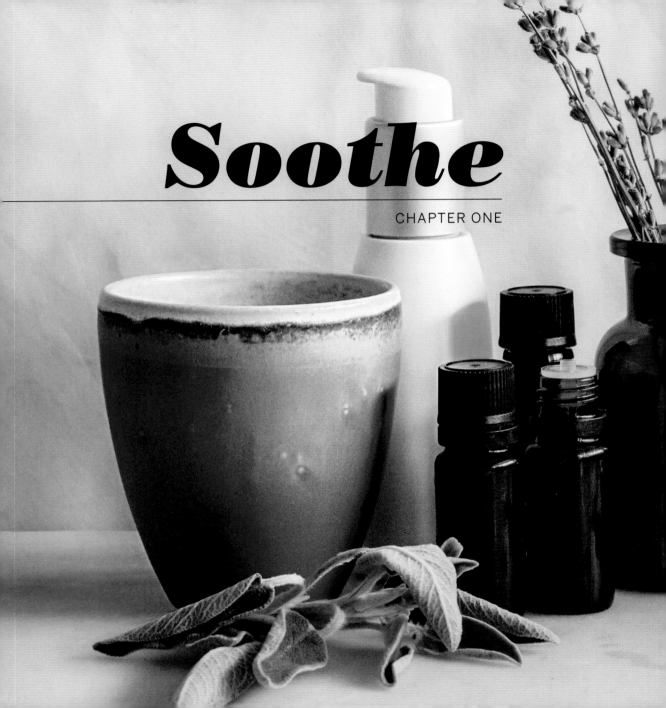

Soothe

CHAPTER ONE

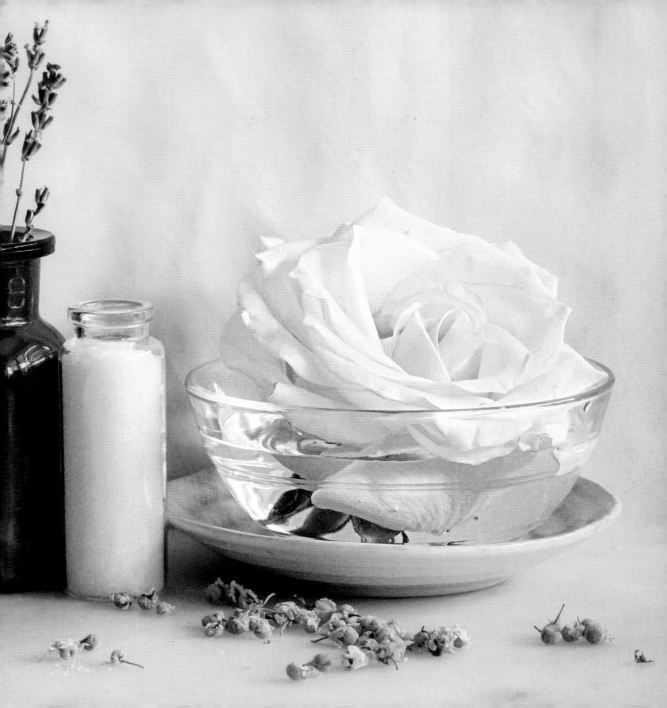

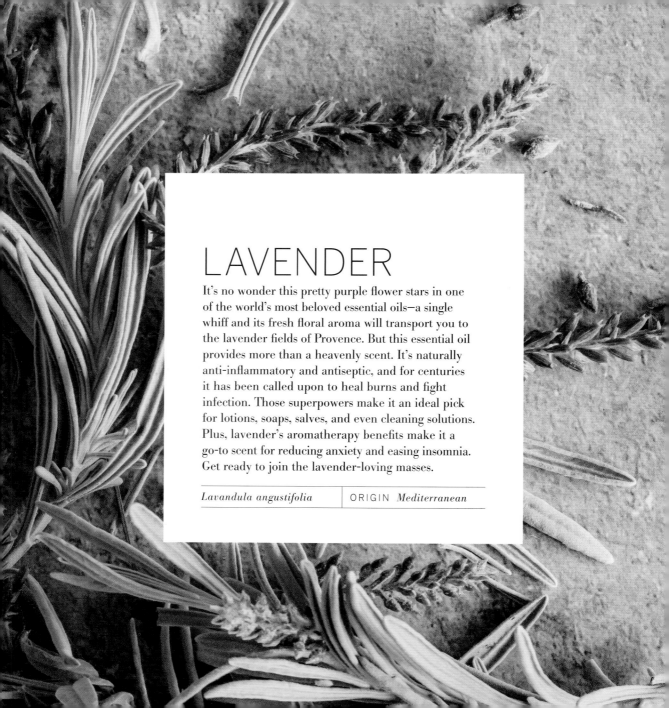

LAVENDER

It's no wonder this pretty purple flower stars in one of the world's most beloved essential oils—a single whiff and its fresh floral aroma will transport you to the lavender fields of Provence. But this essential oil provides more than a heavenly scent. It's naturally anti-inflammatory and antiseptic, and for centuries it has been called upon to heal burns and fight infection. Those superpowers make it an ideal pick for lotions, soaps, salves, and even cleaning solutions. Plus, lavender's aromatherapy benefits make it a go-to scent for reducing anxiety and easing insomnia. Get ready to join the lavender-loving masses.

Lavandula angustifolia | ORIGIN *Mediterranean*

For such a delicately scented essential oil, lavender sure does a lot of heavy lifting around the house. Thanks to its naturally antiseptic properties, it's the perfect candidate for cleansing and refreshing your home—and all without making it reek of the nasty chemicals in store-bought cleaners. Plus, lavender's mood-boosting scent will keep your space full of good vibes.

Lovely Linen Spray

1 cup (240 mL) distilled water

2 tablespoons vodka

40 drops lavender essential oil

10-ounce (295-mL) spray bottle, preferably dark glass

Mix the distilled water, vodka, and lavender essential oil in your spray bottle. Shake well, and voilà—you have a beautifully scented linen spray to keep towels and sheets smelling fresh. The spray will last 1 year; just be sure to shake it before each use.

Scented Fabric Softener

2 cups (475 mL) distilled white vinegar

50 drops lavender essential oil

16-ounce (475-mL) glass jar

Combine the distilled white vinegar with the lavender essential oil in a glass jar. For delicately scented clothes that you'll want to snuggle up in, add ½ cup (120 mL) to the final rinse cycle, or pour it into the fabric softener opening in your washing machine.

Easy All-Purpose Spray Cleaner

¼ cup (60 mL) distilled white vinegar

1½ cups (360 mL) distilled water

1 teaspoon lavender essential oil

16-ounce (475-mL) spray bottle

Gently combine the distilled white vinegar, distilled water, and lavender essential oil in your spray bottle and use as an all-purpose cleaner on just about every surface in your house. Shake the mixture before each use, then spritz the area in need and wipe clean.

Lavender Air Freshener

Pretty bowl of your choice

½ cup (20 g) dried lavender

50 drops lavender essential oil

Fill your chosen bowl with the dried lavender and add in your lavender essential oil. Stir to combine, then place the bowl wherever you like in your home—try the office, nightstand, or bathroom. This refreshing scent will instantly relieve stress and make your space feel like a sanctuary. Refresh with more essential oil after 1 week or as needed.

Lavender + Shea Butter Heel Balm

¼ cup (60 g) beeswax pellets

¼ cup (50 g) shea butter

¼ cup (50 g) coconut oil

¼ cup (60 mL) jojoba oil

50 drops lavender
essential oil

8-ounce (240-mL) jar

It's easy to ignore your feet, but they need just as much TLC as the rest of your skin, especially if you clock major hours standing or make poor footwear choices. Hydrate and heal your heels with this luxurious, rich balm full of ingredients that soothe and repair—including anti-inflammatory and deodorizing lavender.

STEP 1 / In a small heat-safe glass bowl, combine the beeswax, shea butter, coconut oil, and jojoba oil.

STEP 2 / Pour 2 inches (5 cm) of water into a small saucepan and bring it to a boil. Place the bowl over the saucepan and melt the ingredients over low heat, stirring frequently.

STEP 3 / Remove your mixture from the heat and let it cool for 1 minute.

STEP 4 / Add the lavender essential oil and stir gently while the mixture continues to cool.

STEP 5 / Pour the mixture into your jar and allow it to harden completely.

STEP 6 / Slather on this balm nightly before bed to relieve cracked or painful heels. Just be sure to put on socks afterward—unless you like greasy sheets. Use within 6 months.

Anti-Frizz Hair Spritz

1 teaspoon jojoba oil

1 teaspoon vegetable glycerin

2 tablespoons aloe vera gel

10 drops lavender
essential oil

8-ounce (240-mL) spray bottle

6 ounces (180 mL)
distilled water

From the frigid days of winter to summer's moisture-zapping sun, weather sure takes a toll on our tresses. Fight back with this hydrating spray, which contains aloe vera—to condition and nourish your hair—and jojoba and glycerin, which coat the hair strand's outer layer, smoothing the cuticle and reducing frizz.

STEP 1 / Whisk together the jojoba oil, vegetable glycerin, and aloe vera gel in a measuring cup with a spout.

STEP 2 / Drizzle in the lavender essential oil and stir to combine.

STEP 3 / Pour the mixture into your spray bottle. Be sure it has a good pump; if the nozzle is too small, it will get clogged easily.

STEP 4 / Fill the rest of the bottle with distilled water. For best results, refrigerate the bottle when not in use.

STEP 5 / To apply, shake well and spritz onto wet or dry hair from scalp to ends daily. Massage the mixture into your scalp, where the lavender will balance oil production and promote hair growth. Use within 3 months.

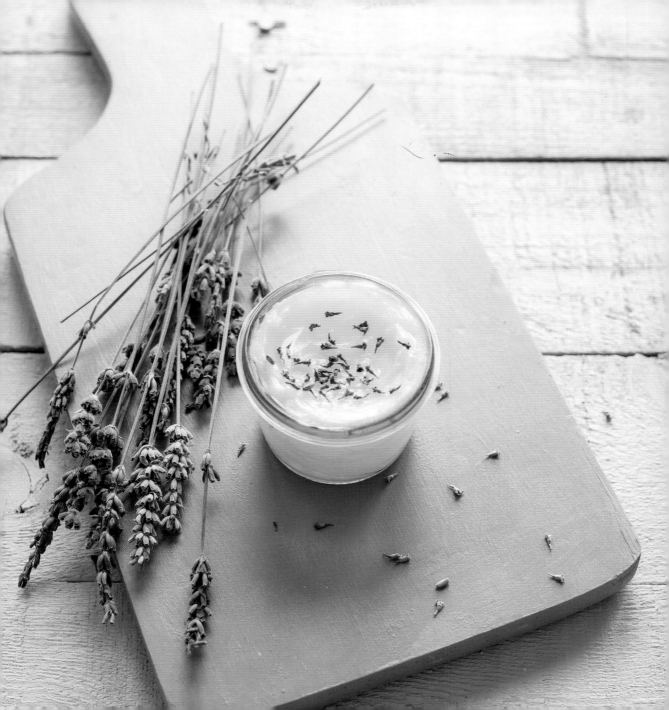

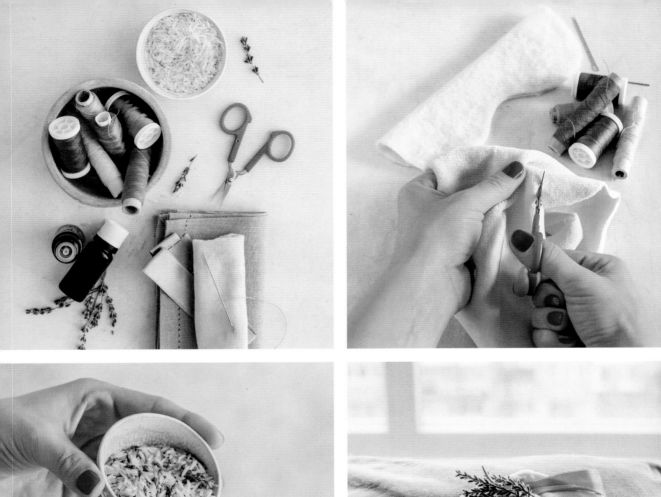
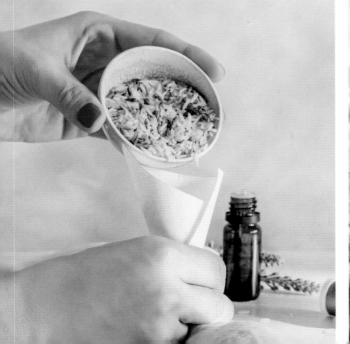
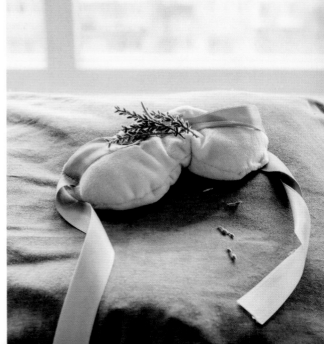

Relaxing Lavender Eye Pillow

18-by-22-inch (46-by-56-cm)
piece of batting

18-by-22-inch (46-by-56-cm)
piece of soft fabric, such as silk
or organic cotton

Scissors

Needle and thread

½ cup (100 g) uncooked
white rice

¼ cup (10 g) dried lavender

15 drops lavender essential oil

Elastic

When I'm feeling overwhelmed, nothing feels better than closing my eyes for just a few minutes to relax my mind and body—and this eye mask does just the trick. Filled with rice and lavender, its soothing scent is perfect for easing a headache or helping you fall asleep. And don't be intimidated by the sewing! It's easy enough to do by hand.

STEP 1 / To start, cut out two sleep mask shapes from the batting. When sewn together, they'll form an interior pouch that will hold the rice and lavender. You can create a template for this mask shape by tracing your favorite pair of sunglasses and adding an extra 1 inch (2.5 cm) for seam allowance.

STEP 2 / Sew the two pieces of batting together around the outside edge, using a ¼-inch (6-mm) seam allowance and leaving a 1- to 2-inch (2.5–5-cm) opening.

STEP 3 / Combine the rice, dried lavender, and lavender essential oil in a bowl and stir.

STEP 4 / Use a funnel to fill the interior pouch with the rice-and-lavender mixture. (You can make a funnel by rolling a sheet of paper into a cone.) Sew the pouch closed.

STEP 5 / Use your template to cut two more sleep mask shapes from the fabric. (Since the mask will rest against your face, make sure to choose a nice, soft fabric—try silk or organic cotton.)

STEP 6 / Cut a length of elastic that fits snugly around the back of your head from temple to temple. Then, with one fabric sleep mask facing right side up, baste (loosely sew together) the ends of the elastic to each side of the mask.

STEP 7 / Position the two fabric sleep masks with right sides facing each other. Sew the masks together with the elastic ends sandwiched between the two masks, leaving a 2-inch (5-cm) opening. Backstitch (reinforce the seam with overlapping stitches) to secure the opening.

STEP 8 / Turn the empty fabric right side out, then stuff the batting pouch inside. Sew the pouch closed.

STEP 9 / Your sleep mask is now ready to wear. To reap the relaxing benefits of the lavender, first warm the mask in the microwave for a few seconds. Always make sure it's not too hot before placing it on your skin.

ROMAN CHAMOMILE

You likely know this botanical as the key ingredient in bedtime tea, and you're not alone: We drink more than 1 million cups of chamomile tea every day. Why so popular? Its dainty blooms contain terpenoids and flavonoids—special chemical compounds that treat everything from allergies and insomnia to wounds and PMS. These miracle-workers also repair irritated skin, which is why chamomile essential oil is a mainstay in creams, soaps, and perfumes. Plus, it's gentle enough to use with children—try it out next time you have an anxious little one on your hands.

| *Chamaemelum nobile* | ORIGIN *Western Europe* |

Wrinkle-Zapping Sheet Mask

1 green tea bag

1 egg white

1 tablespoon honey

3 drops Roman chamomile essential oil

2 two-ply tissues

Try this at-home mask to plump up wrinkles and calm redness. Honey, a humectant that restores moisture, works with chamomile to relieve irritation, while green tea delivers free radical–fighting antioxidants, and the egg tightens and tones fine lines. Use a premade reusable mask or fashion your own with tissues.

STEP 1 / Brew 1 cup (240 mL) green tea and let it cool completely. Pour ¼ cup (60 mL) into a small bowl.

STEP 2 / Add the egg white and honey, and whip with a fork until the egg foams a bit. Then stir in the Roman chamomile essential oil.

STEP 3 / Gingerly pull the two-ply tissues apart and tear each in half.

Soak three of the four pieces in the bowl until they absorb the liquid. (They'll shrink a bit.)

STEP 4 / Layer the three tissue strips across your face. Let them sit for 15 minutes to allow the ingredients to soak into your skin.

STEP 5 / Remove the mask pieces and rinse your face with warm water.

Sleepytime Bubble Bath

¼ cup (60 mL) mild liquid dishwashing soap

½ cup (120 mL) distilled water

¼ cup (60 mL) vegetable glycerin

1 teaspoon Roman chamomile essential oil prediluted in jojoba oil

1 teaspoon pure vanilla extract

10-ounce (295-mL) plastic squirt bottle

It can be a challenge to get kids excited about bath time, but luring them with bubbles is a surefire winner. This bubble bath is easy to make and safe on sensitive skin. Add in Roman chamomile essential oil and vanilla extract to ease restlessness, and get your kids—and yourself—ready for dreamland.

STEP 1 / Combine the liquid dishwashing soap, distilled water, and vegetable glycerin in a spouted measuring cup. (The glycerin helps counteract the drying effects of the soap. You can substitute your favorite carrier oil if you prefer.)

STEP 2 / Add the Roman chamomile essential oil and vanilla extract. Stir gently to combine—you don't want to create a lot of bubbles just yet.

STEP 3 / Pour the mixture into your plastic bottle. (You can go with glass, but plastic is best if you're storing it in the bathroom, where things can get slippery.)

STEP 4 / To use, squirt about 2 tablespoons under running water and agitate to make bubbles. (Note that it won't create enormous foam like the commercial stuff does.) Use within 6 months.

Easy DIY Reed Diffuser

5 to 8 reeds, twigs, or
bamboo skewers

3-ounce (90-mL) or larger
glass bottle

¼ cup (60 mL) light carrier oil,
such as almond or jojoba

20 drops Roman chamomile
essential oil

10 drops ylang ylang
essential oil

5 drops lavender essential oil

Tired of headache-inducing, sickly sweet scented candles and air fresheners? Try this simple yet elegant reed diffuser, which draws up fragrance from a vessel of diluted essential oils and gently releases them into the air. It also comes together in a matter of minutes, and you can customize your blend to suit the room's purpose. This one—which is mainly Roman chamomile—is great for bedrooms.

STEP 1 / Diffuser reeds can be bought online or at a craft store, but if you happen to have bamboo skewers, those work too—just cut off and discard the sharp ends. You can also forage up a rustic array of twigs, as shown here.

STEP 2 / Clean your glass bottle and make sure it's completely dry. (Narrow-neck bottles work best. Search thrift stores for a unique one!)

STEP 3 / Pour the carrier oil into the bottle. (Adjust the ratio accordingly if you're using a larger bottle.)

STEP 4 / Add the chamomile, ylang ylang, and lavender essential oils; stir well to combine.

STEP 5 / Insert the reeds into the bottle. Use as many as will fit into the opening without sticking together; they need room to release the scent.

STEP 6 / Let the reeds sit in the oil blend for between 1 and 2 hours, then turn them over to expose their oil-soaked ends to oxygen.

STEP 7 / Flip over the reeds every couple of days to refresh the scent.

AROMATHERAPY BLENDS FOR YOUR DIFFUSER

Now that you've got your reed diffuser, pick the mix you'd like to have wafting through your home.
WAKE-ME-UP COMBO 15 drops each lemon and peppermint.
ODOR ATTACKER 10 drops each tea tree, lemon, sweet orange, and frankincense, or 10 drops each rosemary, tea tree, lemon, and cinnamon bark.

HAPPY CLEAN COMBO 10 drops each lemon, orange, and grapefruit.
JUST BREATHE 10 drops each bergamot, ylang ylang, and patchouli, or 15 drops each frankincense and bergamot.
RESPIRATORY BLEND 8 drops each rosemary, clove bud, eucalyptus, and cinnamon.

CONCENTRATION BLEND 15 drops each peppermint and sweet orange, or 12 drops lemon and 8 drops each rosemary and cypress.
WIND DOWN 15 drops each lavender and vanilla.
STRESS RELIEVER 10 drops each geranium, bergamot, and lavender.

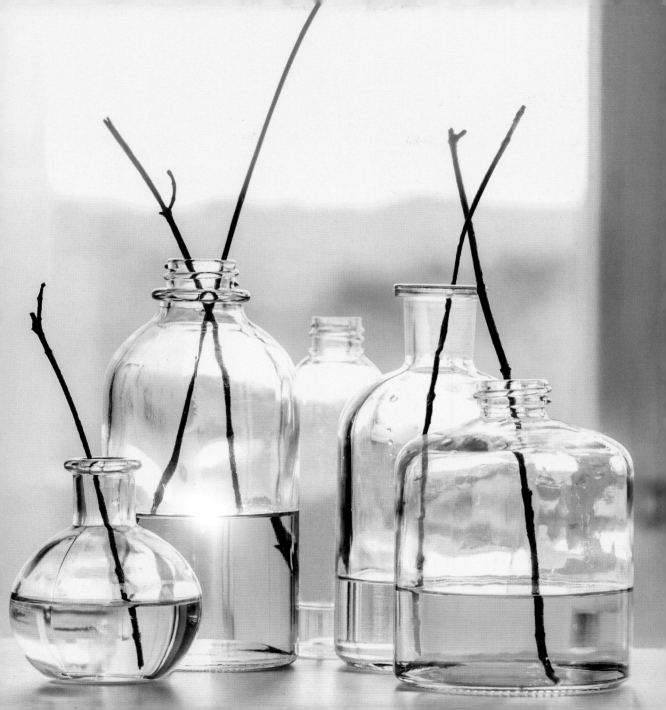

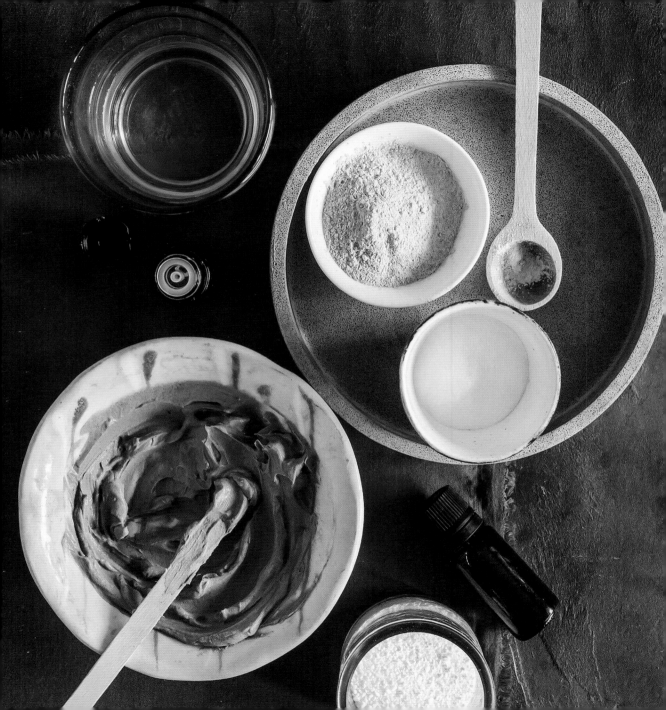

Calming Calamine Lotion

1 tablespoon sea salt

1 tablespoon baking soda

1 tablespoon bentonite clay

Water or witch hazel

10 drops Roman chamomile essential oil

5 drops lavender essential oil

If you're favored by mosquitoes (lucky you!), you don't need a drugstore cream to relieve that itch. Making your own calamine lotion with skin-soothing Roman chamomile essential oil, baking soda, and clay is far less expensive and won't turn you pink. Bentonite clay draws out the sting, while chamomile's anti-inflammatory and pain-relieving properties relieve dry, tingling skin.

STEP 1 / Combine the sea salt, baking soda, and bentonite clay in a small glass or wooden bowl. (Avoid using metal measuring spoons and tools when working with clay, as it will reduce the clay's effectiveness.)

STEP 2 / Slowly add in the water or witch hazel until a paste forms. Either liquid will work fine; witch hazel just happens to have extra cooling and astringent properties, which may prove especially soothing.

STEP 3 / Drizzle in the Roman chamomile and lavender essential oils. Stir to combine completely.

STEP 4 / Apply immediately and liberally to bug bites for instant relief.

Skin-Soothing Diaper Cream

½ cup (100 g) coconut oil

2 tablespoons dried chamomile

¼ cup (50 g) shea butter

1 teaspoon beeswax pellets

18 drops Roman chamomile essential oil

2 tablespoons bentonite clay

8-ounce (240-mL) glass jar

Survive the diaper years with this whipped cream that doubles as a moisturizer for mom's dry hands. With its anti-inflammatory chamomile and superabsorbent bentonite clay, your babies (and their buns) will thank you.

STEP 1 / Bring 2 inches (5 cm) of water to a boil in a small saucepan. Reduce the heat to low and melt the coconut oil in a heat-safe glass bowl set over the saucepan.

STEP 2 / Add the dried chamomile and simmer for 1 hour. Strain and return the infused oil to the bowl.

STEP 3 / Add the shea butter and beeswax pellets. Place the bowl over the saucepan to melt the ingredients.

STEP 4 / Remove the bowl from the heat and let cool for 1 minute, then stir in the Roman chamomile essential oil. Refrigerate until solid.

STEP 5 / Use an immersion blender or hand mixer to whip the mixture until creamy, then stir in the bentonite clay with a wooden spoon.

STEP 6 / Transfer to your jar. Apply liberally to soothe and protect baby bums. Use within 6 months.

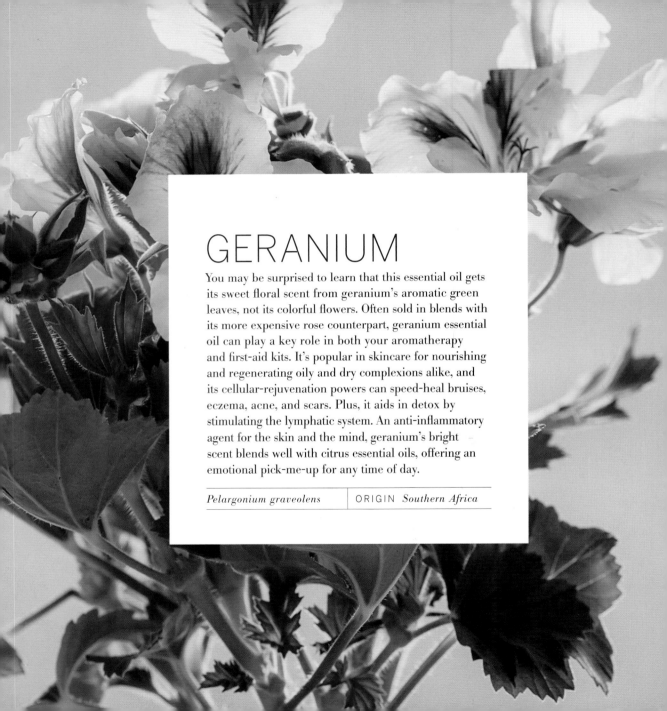

GERANIUM

You may be surprised to learn that this essential oil gets its sweet floral scent from geranium's aromatic green leaves, not its colorful flowers. Often sold in blends with its more expensive rose counterpart, geranium essential oil can play a key role in both your aromatherapy and first-aid kits. It's popular in skincare for nourishing and regenerating oily and dry complexions alike, and its cellular-rejuvenation powers can speed-heal bruises, eczema, acne, and scars. Plus, it aids in detox by stimulating the lymphatic system. An anti-inflammatory agent for the skin and the mind, geranium's bright scent blends well with citrus essential oils, offering an emotional pick-me-up for any time of day.

Pelargonium graveolens | ORIGIN *Southern Africa*

Bump-Be-Gone Shaving Cream

½ cup (100 g) solid coconut oil

¼ cup (60 mL) honey

¼ cup (60 mL) unscented liquid castile soap

2 tablespoons aloe vera gel

48 drops geranium essential oil

24 drops tea tree essential oil

16-ounce (475-mL) plastic container

Why bother to shave your legs if you're rewarded with razor bumps? Add in piping hot water and you've got a recipe for irritated skin. Break the cycle with this DIY shaving cream; its aloe vera and coconut oil make it so rich that shaving won't feel like a thankless chore. The geranium and tea tree essential oils give it a subtle scent too—a far cry from the fake fragrances of store-bought versions.

STEP 1 / In a small bowl, whip the coconut oil with an electric mixer until it's fluffy and smooth. (An immersion blender makes this a snap.)

STEP 2 / With the mixer on low, drizzle in the honey, unscented liquid castile soap, aloe vera gel, and geranium and tea tree essential oils. Whip until the mixture is thoroughly blended, then transfer the cream to your plastic container.

STEP 3 / To get the best shave possible, apply the cream toward the end of your shower, a few minutes before you pick up your razor. Letting it soak in will soften the hair follicles and nourish the skin.

TIP / The shaving cream keeps at room temperature for 4 to 6 months. If you're worried about it going bad, cut the recipe in half or store it in the fridge between uses.

Razor Burn Relief Spray

2 teaspoons jojoba oil

10 drops geranium essential oil

8 drops lavender essential oil

8 drops sandalwood essential oil

5-ounce (150-mL) spray bottle

¼ cup (60 mL) aloe vera gel

¼ cup (60 mL) witch hazel

Razor burn and ingrown hairs usually pop up in spots that get a lot of friction (I'm talking to you, bikini line), which make them especially uncomfortable. Mist those sensitive areas with this aftershave—a cooling treat for red, irritated skin.

STEP 1 / Combine the jojoba oil with the geranium, lavender, and sandalwood essential oils in the spray bottle. Swirl to combine.

STEP 2 / Add the aloe vera gel and witch hazel. Replace the bottle's cap and shake to mix.

STEP 3 / Spritz onto freshly shaved legs and underarms to moisturize the skin, heal irritation, and soothe itchiness. Use within 6 months.

TIP / If you're prone to ingrown hairs, create a gentle scrub by combining 1 tablespoon of this spray with 1 tablespoon sugar. (Add a bit more aloe vera gel if the mixture is too liquid.) Apply to your bikini line to exfoliate blocked pores and fight bacteria; avoid sensitive areas.

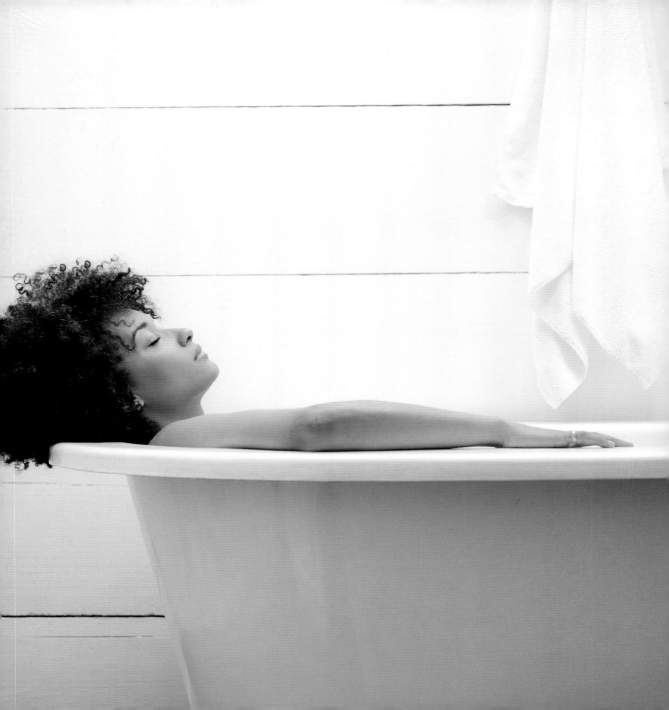

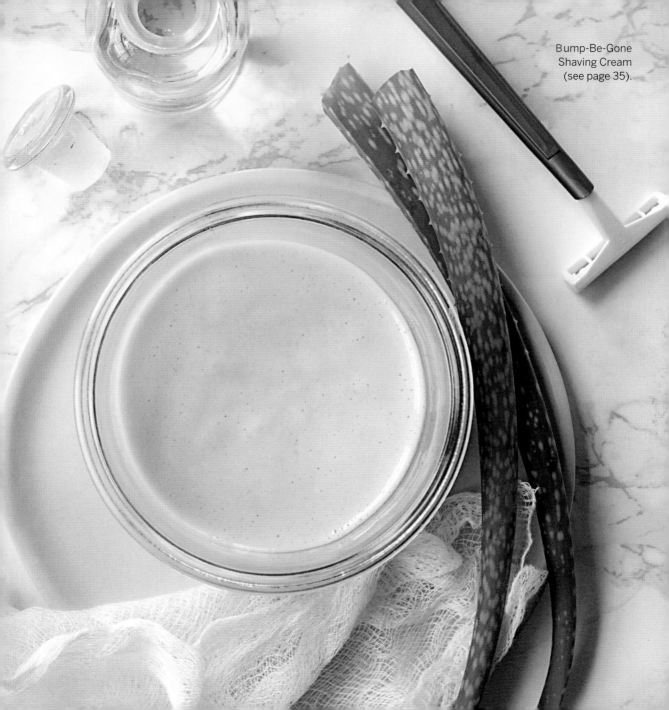

Bump-Be-Gone
Shaving Cream
(see page 35).

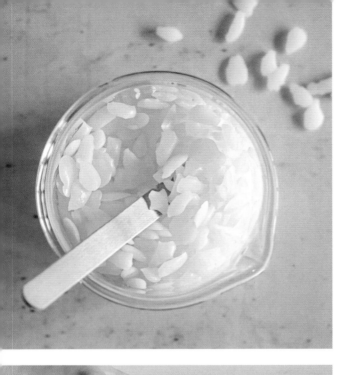

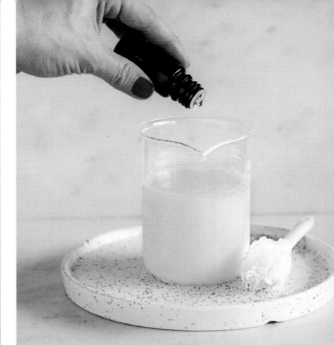

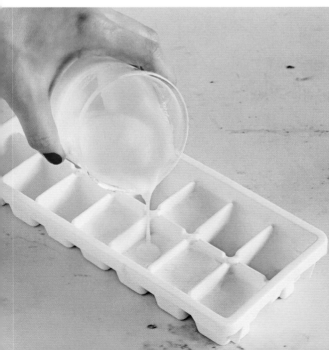

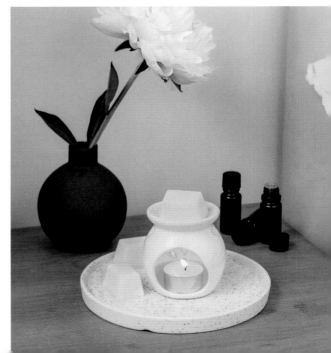

Insect-Repellent Citronella Diffuser Cubes

4 ounces (120 g) pure beeswax (chopped if using bars)

2 tablespoons coconut oil

14 drops geranium essential oil

12 drops citronella essential oil

12 drops rosemary essential oil

10 drops eucalyptus essential oil

Mold, such as an ice cube tray

Candle diffuser

24-ounce (710-mL) airtight container

Forget stinky, oily citronella candles and that gross bug-spray smell! These easy-to-make diffuser cubes do the trick without the overpowering chemical scent. The best part is that the wax never evaporates, so these can be used over and over again (just add more essential oils as needed).

STEP 1 / Heat 2 inches (5 cm) of water in a saucepan until boiling.

STEP 2 / Place the beeswax in a spouted heat-safe glass measuring cup and set it in the saucepan. Turn the dial to medium heat, stirring occasionally, until the beeswax has melted. This can take between 10 and 15 minutes. (Or melt it in the microwave or in a double boiler.)

STEP 3 / Add the coconut oil and stir well to combine it with the wax.

STEP 4 / Remove the cup from the heat and let the mixture cool for 2 to 3 minutes.

STEP 5 / Add the geranium, citronella, rosemary, and eucalyptus essential oils, then stir and pour into a mold. Depending on the size of the mold's wells, you should get six to eight small cubes. Place the mold in the freezer so the wax sets quickly.

STEP 6 / To use, place one cube in the top of a candle diffuser and light it outside. After 10 to 15 minutes, the wax will melt and start diffusing the essential oils. If the scent isn't strong enough or begins to dissipate, just add 2 to 3 more drops of each oil.

STEP 7 / Store the cubes in an airtight container someplace cool and dry. Use within 6 months.

TIP / Be careful when handling the diffuser—it gets very hot. When finished using, allow it to stand until completely cool before handling. To remove any built-up wax, place the cooled diffuser bowl in the fridge or freezer for a few minutes, then pop out the set wax.

Think of these four simple recipes as your starter DIY skincare regimen, and consider geranium essential oil the superstar ingredient in it—no matter what your skin type. This stuff regulates high oil levels, helps reduce the inflammation of acne, and provides crucial moisture and rejuvenation to dry or aging skin.

Balancing + Cleansing Balm

½ teaspoon beeswax pellets

2 tablespoons jojoba oil

1 teaspoon coconut oil

2 teaspoons bentonite clay

1 teaspoon baking soda (optional)

6 drops geranium essential oil

2-ounce (60-mL) container

Melt the beeswax in a spouted heat-safe glass measuring cup in the microwave. Add the jojoba and coconut oils, then use a wooden spoon to stir in the bentonite clay, baking soda (for exfoliation), and geranium essential oil. Transfer to your container. To use, rub a tiny amount into the skin; remove with a soft, wet cloth. Use within 6 months.

Geranium-Lavender Toner

½ cup (120 mL) distilled water

¼ cup (60 mL) witch hazel

1 tablespoon apple cider vinegar

24 drops geranium essential oil

12 drops lavender essential oil

8-ounce (240-mL) bottle

Pour the distilled water, witch hazel, apple cider vinegar, and geranium and lavender essential oils into your bottle, then shake to combine. Apply to your face with a cotton pad in between cleansing and moisturizing. Be sure to use this recipe within 3 months.

Easy Everyday Facial Oil

2 tablespoons jojoba oil

8 drops geranium essential oil

4 drops frankincense essential oil

1-ounce (30-mL) dark glass jar

For a simple daily moisturizer for all skin types, mix the jojoba oil with the geranium and frankincense essential oils in a dark glass jar. Apply 2 to 4 drops to skin after cleansing and toning; use within 3 months.

Hydrating Honey Mask

1 teaspoon vitamin E oil (about 8 capsules)

2 drops geranium essential oil

¼ avocado, smashed

1 teaspoon honey

Mix the vitamin E oil and geranium essential oil in a small bowl with the smashed avocado and honey. Apply weekly to your face and neck. Leave on for 10 to 15 minutes, then rinse off with warm water and follow up with moisturizer. Use within 3 months.

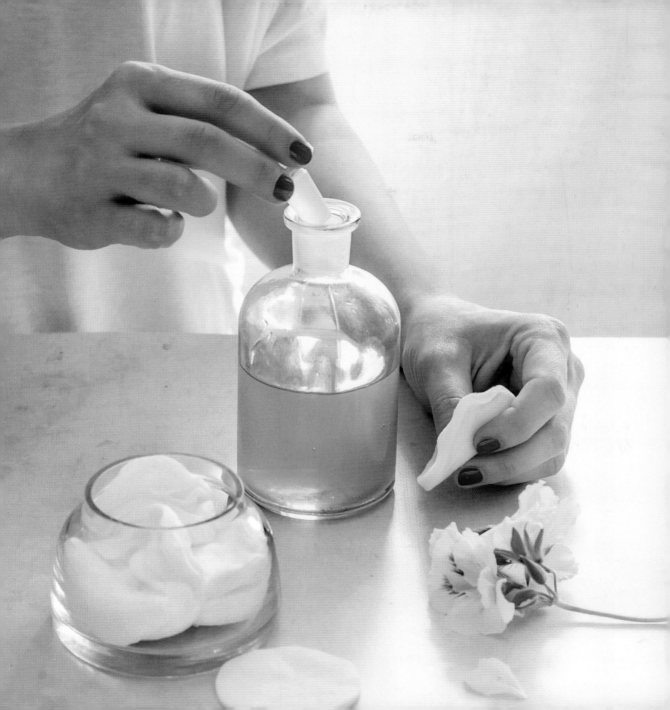

Meditation

Meditation not only relaxes the body, it also quiets the mind and calms the nervous system. So switch off the TV, turn your phone to silent, and shut the door. Then use these simple and soothing essential oil blends to create a relaxed, peaceful environment that lets you fully unplug from the world.

SWITCH-IT-UP ELECTRIC ROOM DIFFUSION

To mix up your blends daily (or even hourly), pick up an electric diffuser, and load it up with specific blends that help you meditate on whatever's on your mind. Scale the volume per your diffuser's instructions.

Geranium
3 drops

Anise
2 drops

Roman
Chamomile
2 drops

Myrtle
3 drops

QUICK-SPRITZ GROUNDING YOGA SPRAY

Make your practice to go with a portable blend. Pour the below mix of essential oils with 4 ounces (120 mL) water into a travel-size spray bottle, and spritz to get your om on when you travel. Shake well before use.

Frankincense
50 drops

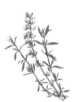

Hyssop
50 drops

Lemon
50 drops

SERENITY ROLL-ON PERFUME

This discreet scent comes to your rescue whenever you need a little mindfulness. Combine this 10-drop blend in a 10-mL roll-on applicator and top it off with carrier oil. Apply to your wrists, upper chest, and the back of your neck.

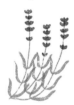

Lavender
4 drops

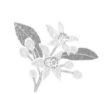

Neroli
3 drops

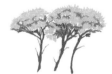

Helichrysum
3 drops

CALMING MASSAGE OIL

Up your rubdown's meditative powers by adding this simple essential oil ratio to 6 teaspoons of a carrier oil of your choosing, such as sweet almond, jojoba, apricot kernel, or coconut.

Vetiver
6 drops

Sweet Marjoram
5 drops

Lavender
5 drops

Atlas Cedarwood
4 drops

MINI-VACATION BODY SPRAY

Transport yourself to more relaxing climes with a blend of 3 tablespoons coconut water, 2 teaspoons aloe vera gel, and this essential oil mix. Keep in a 2-ounce (60-mL) spray bottle and mist when the need arises.

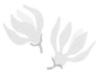
Sweet Orange
6 drops

Ylang Ylang
6 drops

Palmarosa
8 drops

Lime
4 drops

DREAMY REED DIFFUSER

For a decorative display that reminds you to fit a little zen into your daily life, mix these essential oils together with ¼ cup (60 mL) carrier oil in a small bottle. Stick 5 to 8 reeds into the mixture to subtly scent the air.

Clary Sage
16 drops

Atlas Cedarwood
16 drops

Neroli
8 drops

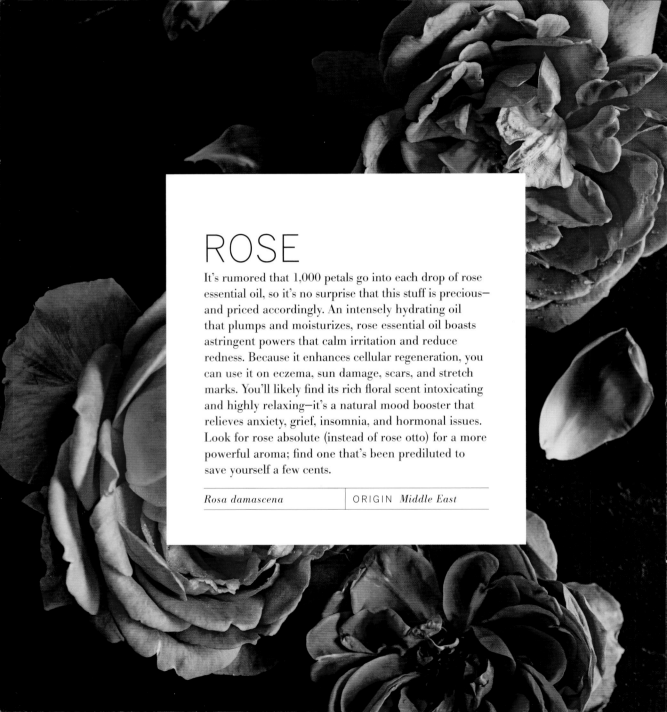

ROSE

It's rumored that 1,000 petals go into each drop of rose essential oil, so it's no surprise that this stuff is precious—and priced accordingly. An intensely hydrating oil that plumps and moisturizes, rose essential oil boasts astringent powers that calm irritation and reduce redness. Because it enhances cellular regeneration, you can use it on eczema, sun damage, scars, and stretch marks. You'll likely find its rich floral scent intoxicating and highly relaxing—it's a natural mood booster that relieves anxiety, grief, insomnia, and hormonal issues. Look for rose absolute (instead of rose otto) for a more powerful aroma; find one that's been prediluted to save yourself a few cents.

Rosa damascena | ORIGIN *Middle East*

Flower Power Deodorant

2 tablespoons vodka
(the higher the proof, the better)

2 tablespoons distilled water

2-ounce (60-mL) dark glass
spray bottle

3 drops rose essential oil

2 drops jasmine
essential oil

2 drops sweet orange
essential oil

1 drop lavender essential oil

No, you're not mixing up a vodka cocktail—it's a delightful DIY deodorant spray with powerful (but not overpowering) floral notes. Don't skip the booze, as it's essential for dispersing the oils and helping the scent linger longer in the pit area. It also slows down the sweat factor, keeping you dry and fresh-smelling all day.

STEP 1 / Pour the vodka and distilled water into your dark spray bottle. (The dark glass will protect the essential oils from light, preventing degradation and lengthening the spray's shelf life.)

STEP 2 / Drizzle in the rose, jasmine, sweet orange, and lavender essential oils. Screw on the lid and shake well to combine.

STEP 3 / Before each use, agitate the bottle to redistribute the oils. Give each underarm 2 to 3 spritzes and let your pits air-dry. It might sting for a second if you've just shaved. Apply again after exercise or perspiration, or simply whenever you want to enjoy the sweet floral smell. For best results, use within 3 months.

Serene Magnesium Mist

¼ cup (60 mL) rose water

2 tablespoons Epsom salt

2-ounce (60-mL) spray bottle

18 drops rose essential oil

12 drops sandalwood
essential oil

There's nothing like an Epsom salt bath to ease nerves and soothe sore muscles. But why limit this wonder-worker to the tub? Try it in a gentle spray to absorb the natural magnesium whenever you like; it will combat insomnia, stress, and depression. Diluted with aromatic rose water, this mist gets a boost from rose and sandalwood essential oils, which can help you find calm in times of change.

STEP 1 / Add the rose water to a small saucepan; warm over low heat. Stir in the Epsom salt.

STEP 2 / Remove the mixture from the heat and let it cool. Pour it into your spray bottle.

STEP 3 / Add the rose and sandalwood essential oils, screw on the top, and shake to combine.

STEP 4 / To use, spray onto your arms, legs, or abdomen, then gently rub it in. Post-shower is the perfect time for this treatment—before you apply any other products—but you can mist your skin up to 6 times a day. If you experience any skin irritation, rinse off immediately. Use within 3 months.

Luxurious Rose Milk Bath

1½ cups (190 g) full-fat powdered milk

½ cup (120 g) Epsom salt

2 drops natural red food coloring (optional)

¼ cup (5 g) dried rose petals

5 drops rose essential oil

Decorative bottle or sachet

This pretty-in-pink milk bath requires hardly any effort beyond finding a cute jar to store it in. The rose petals and essential oil make the bathwater smell divine (and ease stress and depression), while the Epsom salt draws out toxins from the body, relaxes muscles, and loosens stiff joints. Package it up in a small bottle or sachet as a present for a hard-working lady in your life.

STEP 1 / Combine the skin-softening powdered milk and Epsom salt in a mixing bowl.

STEP 2 / Add the natural food coloring and stir until the mixture is uniformly pink. (You can skip the food coloring, but I love the pretty hue.)

STEP 3 / Add the dried rose petals and rose essential oil. Stir the mixture again to combine the ingredients.

STEP 4 / Pour the milk bath into a bottle or sachet. To enjoy, add ½ cup (70 g) of the mixture to a warm bath. Use within 6 months.

Petal + Oats Face Scrub

1 tablespoon dried rose petals

1 tablespoon dried chamomile

1 tablespoon old-fashioned oats

2-ounce (60-mL) container

1 tablespoon full-fat powdered milk

3 drops rose essential oil

Water, honey, or yogurt

Exfoliating is like flossing: We know it's important, but that doesn't mean we do it enough. Whip up this amazing scrub, however, and you'll soon look forward to your weekly buffing routine. Rose petals are full of malic and citric acids—which slough off dead cells, clearing the way for healthy ones—while chamomile calms irritated skin. The rose essential oil helps plump up fine lines and reduce redness.

STEP 1 / Combine the dried rose petals and chamomile with the old-fashioned oats in a coffee grinder; pulse until finely ground.

STEP 2 / Transfer the mixture to a sealable container (such as a small mason jar). Add the powdered milk and the rose essential oil, then stir the ingredients together.

STEP 3 / To use, mix 1 teaspoon of the dry mixture with water, honey, or yogurt to form a paste. Apply as a mask immediately after cleansing your face, then scrub away after 10 minutes using a circular motion.

STEP 4 / Rinse with warm water, then finish with toner and moisturizer. Keep sealed and completely dry. Use within 6 months.

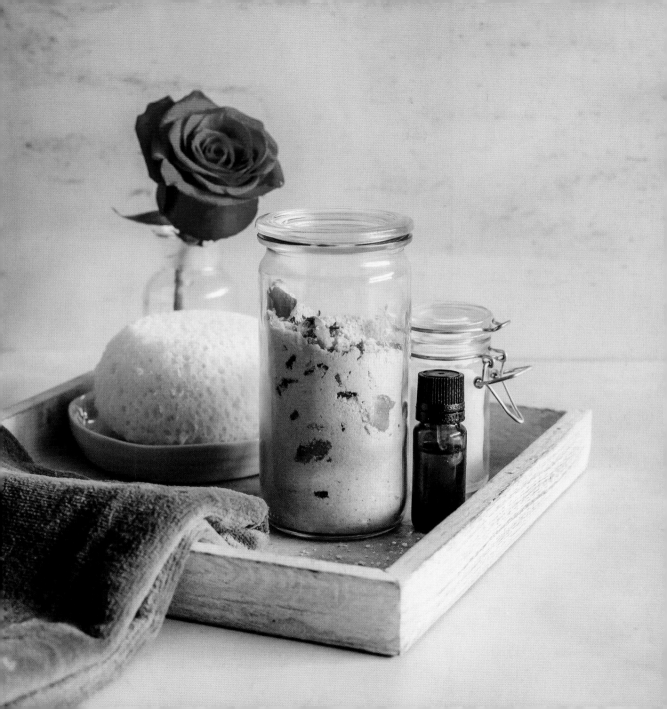

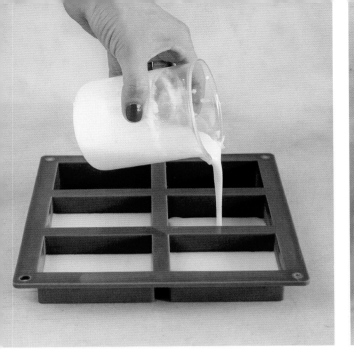

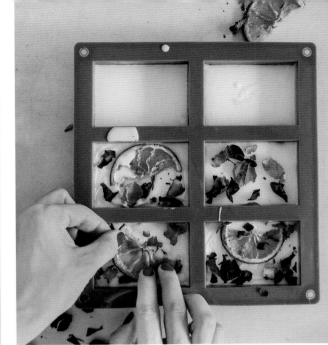

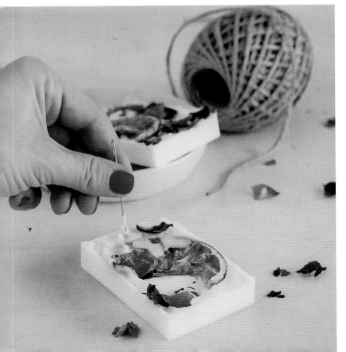

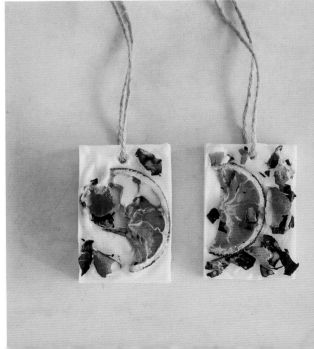

Pretty Floral Wax Sachets

2 cups (180 g) soy wax flakes

1 teaspoon rose absolute oil prediluted in jojoba oil

1 teaspoon sweet orange essential oil

½ cup (10 g) dried rose petals or buds

6 to 10 dried orange slices

Silicone mold

Long metal nail (or thick needle)

Twine, string, or ribbon

Wax sachets are the best of both worlds: They smell as wonderful as candles, but you'll never forget to blow them out! You can make these lovely bars in a single afternoon, then set them wherever you like: on your desk or in the bathroom, or in a window where the sun can warm the wax and release its fragrance. You can even hang them in your closet to delicately scent your clothes.

STEP 1 / Fill a spouted heat-safe glass measuring cup or a clean aluminum soup can with 1½ cups (135 g) soy wax flakes.

STEP 2 / Place the container in the center of a small saucepan. Add water to the saucepan until it reaches halfway up the container's sides.

STEP 3 / Bring the water to a boil over medium heat and keep a watchful eye on the wax until it's completely melted. As it melts, continue adding the remaining flakes until the container is almost full of liquid wax.

STEP 4 / Carefully remove the container from the water. Let it cool for 1 minute, then add the rose absolute oil and sweet orange essential oil. Stir to combine.

STEP 5 / Arrange half the dried rose petals and citrus slices in the bottom of your silicone mold. Then carefully pour about three-fourths of the wax into the molds to a depth of about ¼ inch (6 mm).

STEP 6 / When the sachets have started to set but are still warm and pliable, press the remaining dried rose petals and citrus pieces into the sachets' surfaces.

STEP 7 / Use a paintbrush to gently apply a thin layer of liquid wax over the botanicals, sealing them in.

STEP 8 / When the wax has cooled completely, gingerly remove the sachets from the molds.

STEP 9 / Take a long metal nail (or thick needle) and cautiously heat it for a few seconds over an open flame. Take care not to burn yourself.

STEP 10 / Use the hot nail to melt a small hole through the tops of your wax bars. (I found it best to start at the back and go through to the front.)

STEP 11 / Thread a piece of twine through the hole and knot it. Hang your wax sachets wherever you want to add scent and a decorative touch.

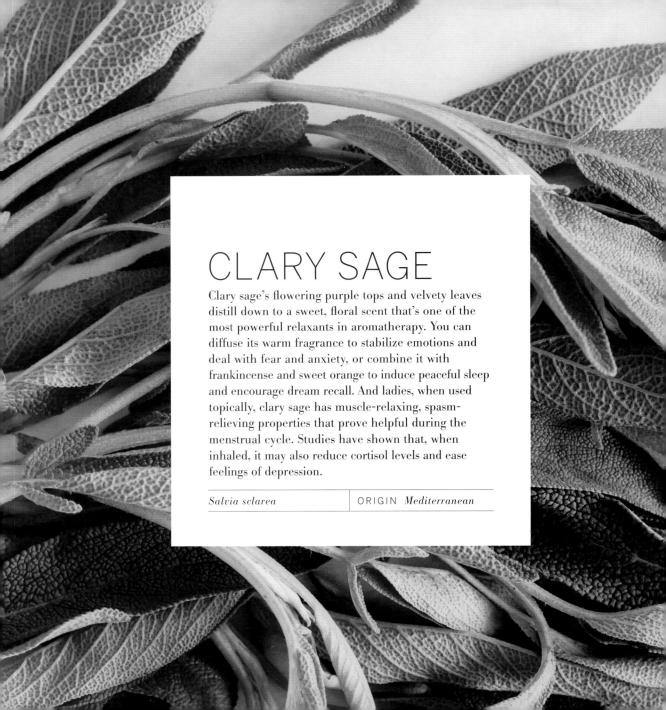

CLARY SAGE

Clary sage's flowering purple tops and velvety leaves distill down to a sweet, floral scent that's one of the most powerful relaxants in aromatherapy. You can diffuse its warm fragrance to stabilize emotions and deal with fear and anxiety, or combine it with frankincense and sweet orange to induce peaceful sleep and encourage dream recall. And ladies, when used topically, clary sage has muscle-relaxing, spasm-relieving properties that prove helpful during the menstrual cycle. Studies have shown that, when inhaled, it may also reduce cortisol levels and ease feelings of depression.

Salvia sclarea   ORIGIN *Mediterranean*

Monthly Breakout Moisturizer

¼ cup (50 g) shea butter
1 teaspoon vitamin E oil
1 teaspoon grape-seed oil
12 drops clary sage essential oil
6 drops thyme essential oil
6 drops sandalwood essential oil
3-ounce (90-mL) glass jar

Along with stress and clogged pores, fluctuating hormones around your period might cause flare-ups on your chin and jaw—even after the teenage years. Clary sage battles acne-causing bacteria, and it also regulates hormones and lowers cortisol levels, which are associated with stress and pesky pimples. Thyme offers an extra pimple-fighting kick while sandalwood combats excess oil.

STEP 1 / Melt the shea butter in a heat-safe glass bowl in the microwave or in a double boiler. You can even soften it in the sun.

STEP 2 / Add the vitamin E and grape-seed oils, then drizzle in the clary sage, thyme, and sandalwood essential oils. Stir well to combine.

STEP 3 / Transfer to your glass jar and replace the lid. (Depending on the temperature, it may thicken to a solid; heat it up before use, if needed.)

STEP 4 / To use, apply a small amount to clean skin each night or during hormonal breakouts. Use it all up within 6 months.

Hormonal Spot Treatment

1-ounce (30-mL) roll-on applicator
8 drops clary sage essential oil
4 drops lavender essential oil
2 drops tea tree essential oil
1 ounce (30 mL) apricot kernel oil

Let this fragrant blend of clary sage and lavender lift you out of the moodiness that can come with hormonal changes. Add tea tree and you've packed in three of the best acne-fighting essential oils. Together they halt bacteria and repair inflamed skin—all while being gentler than over-the-counter treatments.

STEP 1 / Pop the rollerball out of your applicator and add the clary sage, lavender, and tea tree essential oils. Then fill the applicator with apricot kernel oil, which is both anti-inflammatory and antibacterial.

STEP 2 / Replace the rollerball and cap, then shake to combine the oils.

STEP 3 / To use, first roll the bottle between your hands to redistribute the oils. Then roll the treatment onto any breakouts twice a day until healed. The essential oils fight acne as well as work to lighten dark spots and the scars that pimples can leave in their wake. Make sure to use within 6 months.

Sage Smudging Ritual

2 to 3 sprigs fresh or
dried herbs

6 to 8 fresh sage leaves

100 percent cotton twine

4 drops clary sage essential oil

4 drops sandalwood essential oil

2 drops bergamot essential oil

Clearing the air is a must when you're moving into a new house, spring cleaning, or just need some fresh energy in your home. Diffusing a blend of clary sage, sandalwood, and bergamot essential oils will do the trick—especially if you kick-start the purification process with a sage smudging ritual. These little bundles of dried herbs and flowers come to us from various Native American cultures, where sage has long been burned in ceremonies to cleanse and bless.

STEP 1 / Cinch together a few sprigs of any long-stemmed herbs or flowers you have, like roses that have passed their prime or that lavender bush you forgot to water. You can also use small cuttings from pine or cedar trees.

STEP 2 / Wrap this small bouquet in the sage leaves, using as many as you need to cover the bundle.

STEP 3 / Measure and cut a piece of cotton twine about three times as long as your bundle.

STEP 4 / Knot the twine ½ inch (1.25 cm) from the stems' ends. Leave it long on one side and short— 2 inches (5 cm)—on the other.

STEP 5 / Start wrapping the long end of the twine around the bundle. Keep it tight, since the twine will loosen as the herbs dry and shrink. Tuck in any loose ends between the sage leaves as you wind your way up.

STEP 6 / When you reach the end, wind the twine back the other direction, crisscrossing the twine that you just wrapped around the bundle.

STEP 7 / When you reach the bundle's end, tie off the twine. Wrap any extra around the base and tuck in the ends. This creates a nice handle.

STEP 8 / Find a cool, dry spot to hang the bundle, and let it air-dry for 2 to 3 weeks. Make sure the bundle is completely dry before burning.

STEP 9 / When the smudge stick is dry, hold the handle end and light the other one until you get a flame going. Blow out the fire and let the stick smolder. To cleanse yourself, wave the smoke from your feet to your head, then back down again. To smudge your home, walk the smoke into the corners and doorways.

STEP 10 / Let the smudge stick burn out in a small heat-safe bowl and enjoy the calming herbal scent.

STEP 11 / To continue cleansing the air (and remove any lingering smoke scent), add the clary sage, sandalwood, and bergamot essential oils to a diffuser of your choosing and keep the good vibes flowing.

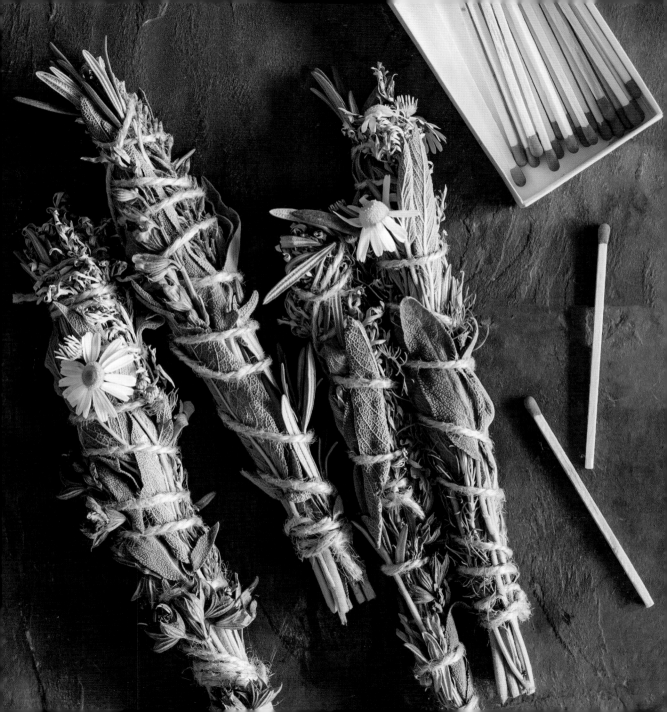

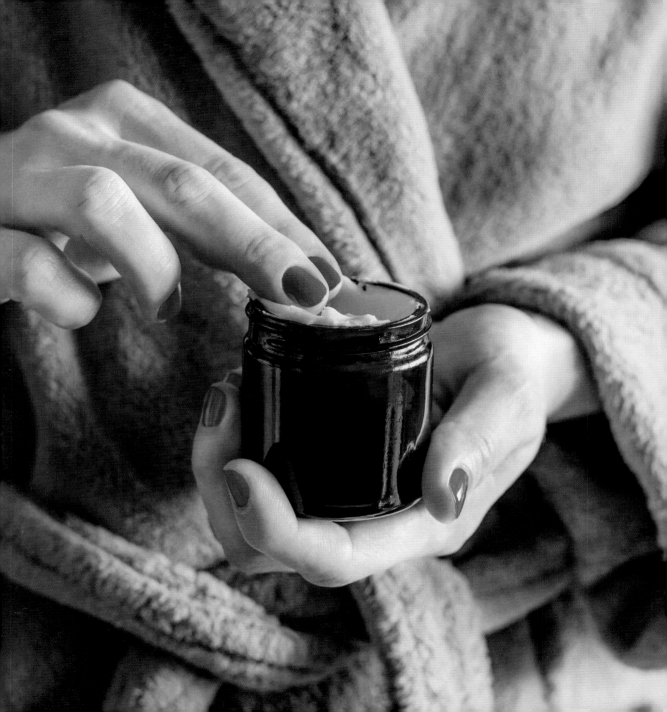

PMS Relief Balm

6 tablespoons raspberry-leaf-infused oil (see page 16)

2 tablespoons beeswax

2 tablespoons evening primrose oil

36 drops clary sage essential oil

36 drops geranium essential oil

25 drops sweet marjoram essential oil

25 drops ginger essential oil

12 drops cinnamon leaf essential oil

5-ounce (150-mL) lidded container

Your first instinct when you have PMS might be to pop a pain pill, grab a heating pad, and head to bed. Instead of masking your symptoms, try this soothing balm, which supports the reproductive system and hormone regulation with clary sage, primrose, and raspberry leaf. Packed with valuable vitamins, magnesium, iron, and potassium, raspberry leaf naturally strengthens and tones the muscles of the uterus. It can ease menstrual cramping—not to mention grumpy moods.

STEP 1 / To start, make raspberry-leaf-infused oil according to the instructions on page 16. (You can also purchase it, if you prefer.)

STEP 2 / Bring 2 inches (5 cm) of water to a low simmer in a small saucepan.

STEP 3 / Put the raspberry-leaf infusion and beeswax in a medium heat-safe glass bowl. Place the bowl over the saucepan.

STEP 4 / When the ingredients have melted, remove the bowl from the heat. Add your evening primrose oil and the clary sage, geranium, sweet marjoram, ginger, and cinnamon leaf essential oils; stir.

STEP 5 / Pour the melted mixture into a clean, dry container and put the lid on. Let it sit until the balm is firm. Keep the finished product in a cool and dry spot.

STEP 6 / Enjoy your balm any time symptoms arise by massaging it directly onto your abdomen and lower back. Use within 8 months.

TIP / This essential oil blend is pretty potent—it's meant to be used a few times a month (not daily) to relieve cramping. Don't have beeswax? Just combine the liquid oils and use as a massage oil.

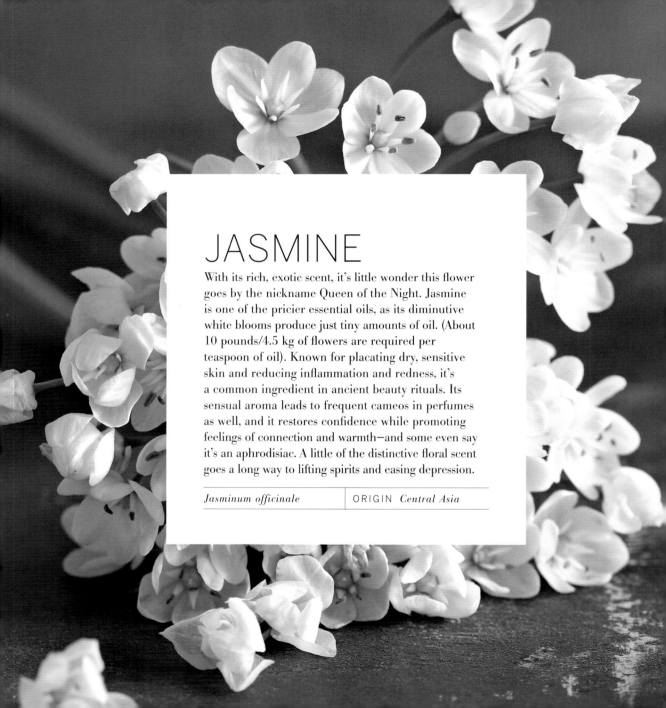

JASMINE

With its rich, exotic scent, it's little wonder this flower goes by the nickname Queen of the Night. Jasmine is one of the pricier essential oils, as its diminutive white blooms produce just tiny amounts of oil. (About 10 pounds/4.5 kg of flowers are required per teaspoon of oil). Known for placating dry, sensitive skin and reducing inflammation and redness, it's a common ingredient in ancient beauty rituals. Its sensual aroma leads to frequent cameos in perfumes as well, and it restores confidence while promoting feelings of connection and warmth—and some even say it's an aphrodisiac. A little of the distinctive floral scent goes a long way to lifting spirits and easing depression.

Jasminum officinale | ORIGIN *Central Asia*

All-Natural Deodorant Bar

2 tablespoons beeswax pellets
¼ cup (50 g) shea butter
¼ cup (50 g) coconut oil
2 tablespoons baking soda
2 tablespoons cornstarch
20 drops jasmine essential oil
10 drops tea tree essential oil
Soap molds
Large container

DIY deodorant is a gamble, but with the right essential oils—in this case, jasmine and tea tree—you'll stay fresh as a daisy. (Or a jasmine blossom, as it were.) In addition to tea tree essential oil's antibacterial and antiviral properties, jasmine relieves bumps and redness (perfect for just-shaved underarms), as well as improves mood, decreases stress, and boosts concentration—three things your current deodorant probably doesn't do.

STEP 1 / Combine the beeswax, shea butter, and coconut oil in a small heat-safe glass bowl. These ingredients will work together to keep your skin feeling smooth to the touch.

STEP 2 / Pour 2 inches (5 cm) of water into a small saucepan and warm it over low heat. Place the glass bowl over the saucepan to gently melt the wax and oils together, stirring frequently. (You can also use a double boiler if you have one.)

STEP 3 / Remove from the heat and stir in the baking soda and cornstarch. These ingredients are the lifesavers that keep you dry.

STEP 4 / Drizzle in the jasmine and tea tree essential oils; mix together.

STEP 5 / Pour the mixture into molds of your choosing. You can find plastic soap molds at craft stores, or you can use ice cube trays, silicone molds, or plastic food storage containers. You can also pour the mixture into deodorant containers just like you find at the drugstore. This recipe will create about 6 ounces (170 g).

STEP 6 / Let the mixture harden at room temperature for several hours. Then gingerly pop the bars out of the molds and store them in a container with a tight-fitting lid. Use within 1 year.

TIP / To make moisturizing lotion bars instead of deodorant bars, simply omit the baking soda and cornstarch.

Jasmine-Aloe Perfume Body Spray

4-ounce (120-mL) spray bottle
Assorted dried flowers
(optional)
Mica flakes (optional)
3 ounces (90 mL) witch hazel
with aloe vera
2 tablespoons vegetable glycerin
25 drops jasmine essential oil

When hot weather calls for lightweight lotions and perfumes, look to this aromatic mist to keep you fresh while also providing nourishment. Plus, its sultry jasmine scent will mentally carry you away to tropical locales and help you unwind. Go with a special witch hazel that includes aloe vera; it will help your skin lock in moisture, which is essential if you've been out in the sun, sand, or sea.

STEP 1 / Fill your spray bottle with the dried flowers and shimmery mica, if using. (These ingredients are just for looks; feel free to skip them if you wish to simplify.)

STEP 2 / Add the aloe-vera-enhanced witch hazel and vegetable glycerin to the spray bottle, then top it off with the jasmine essential oil. Swirl the bottle to combine all the ingredients.

STEP 3 / To use, mist all over when you need a de-stressing refresher. Avoid getting it in your eyes, as the witch hazel will sting! Use within 3 months.

Coconut Oil Stretch Mark Scrub

1 tablespoon shea butter
¼ cup (50 g) coconut oil
½ cup (125 g) organic raw
cane sugar
4 drops jasmine essential oil
2 drops bergamot essential oil
8-ounce (240-mL) glass jar

For most of us, stretch marks are just a fact of life—they're the epidermis's natural response to growth. While there's absolutely nothing wrong with them, this rejuvenating scrub can help minimize their appearance by boosting collagen production and softening the skin.

STEP 1 / Combine the shea butter and coconut oil in a small bowl. If the shea butter is too hard, heat the bowl in the microwave in 5-second blasts until it's soft and malleable.

STEP 2 / Blend in the sugar, then fold in the jasmine and bergamot essential oils.

STEP 3 / Transfer the scrub to your glass jar with a tight-fitting lid, being sure to keep water out of the mixture.

STEP 4 / To use, take a small scoop out of the jar with a dry spoon. Massage into the skin 2 or 3 times per week. Use within 6 months.

TIP / For best results, follow the scrub with this skin-healing balm: Melt ¼ cup (50 g) shea butter and ¼ cup (50 g) coconut oil over low heat, then add 8 drops jasmine essential oil. Let cool before use. Store in a 4-ounce (120-mL) glass jar, and use within 3 months.

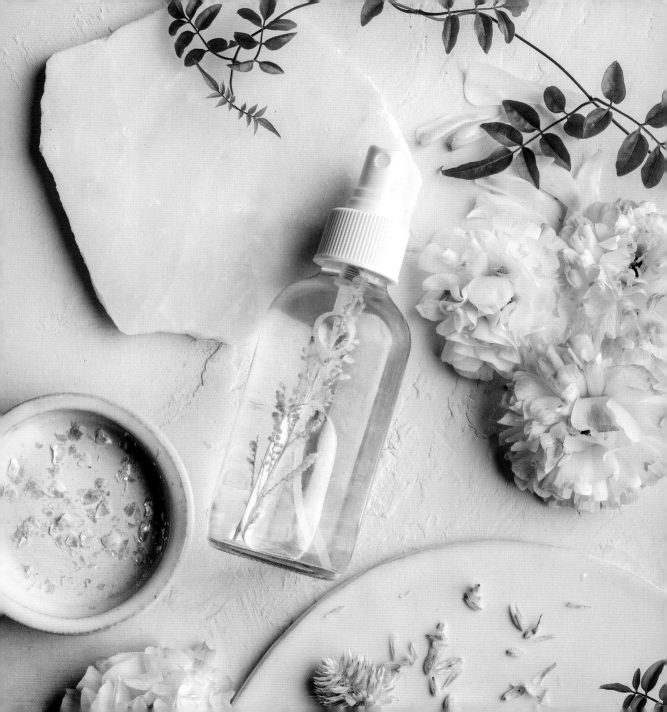

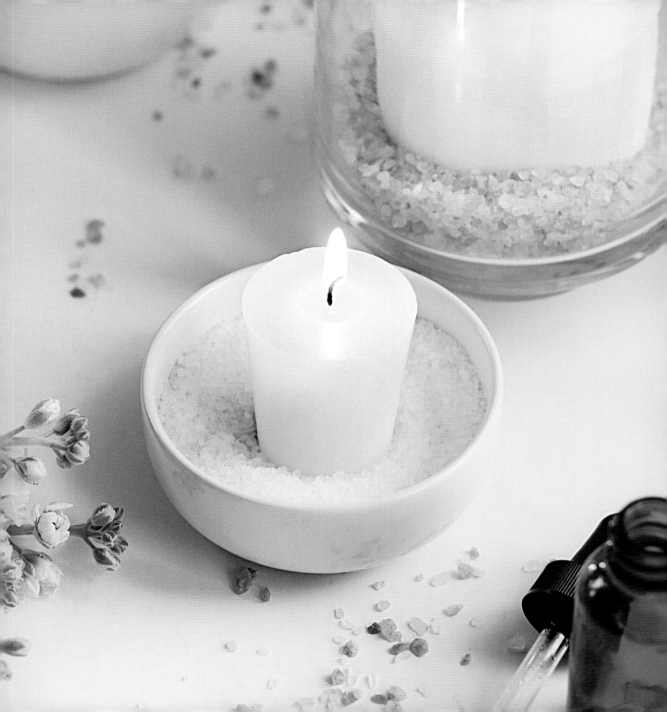

Pink Himalayan Salt Candle Diffuser

1 cup (265 g) pink
Himalayan salt

10 drops jasmine essential oil

6 drops sweet orange
essential oil

4 drops sandalwood essential oil

Unscented votive candles and
candle holders

What's more relaxing than the soft glow of candlelight, especially when paired with the soothing aroma of essential oils? Much like their lamp counterparts, Himalayan salt diffusers cleanse the air of impurities by attracting water vapor— and all the mold, bacteria, and allergens that it carries. This simple homemade model has the added bonus of diffusing essential oils at the same time.

STEP 1 / Pour the salt into a small mixing bowl. If you don't have any pink Himalayan salt on hand, don't worry—any natural sea salt will do. (In fact, I like to set up diffusers of different-colored salts around the house—try red Hawaiian, French gray, or black Nepalese.)

STEP 2 / Drizzle in the jasmine, sweet orange, and sandalwood essential oils. Stir the salts to distribute the oils.

STEP 3 / Place a votive candle in the bottom of a candle holder, glass jar, or small shallow bowl. Pour the

salt around the candle until it reaches halfway up its sides.

STEP 4 / Light the candle and let the heat warm the salts, activating their purifying powers and helping release the essential oils. You can keep indefinitely refreshing the salt with oils as needed.

TIP / Since the sea salt must be warm to purify the air, short votives work better than tall pillar candles, since they burn quicker and bring the heat closer to the salt. Caveat: You'll need to keep a closer eye on them so they don't become a fire hazard.

MORE BLENDS FOR YOUR SALT CANDLE DIFFUSER

Lots of essential oils will work great in a Himalayan salt candle diffuser. Here are some of my favorite blends to diffuse throughout the day. Aim for about 20 drops essential oils for 1 cup (265 g) salt.
RELAXING 10 drops each cedarwood and frankincense.

ENERGIZING 10 drops lemongrass and 5 drops each ylang ylang and sweet orange.
MOOD BOOSTER 10 drops sweet orange and 10 drops each either grapefruit or lemon.
FOCUSING 10 drops each peppermint and rosemary.

DEODORIZING 6 drops each cinnamon, clove bud, and tea tree.
HARMONY 10 drops each cypress and sandalwood.
BUG OFF 5 drops each eucalyptus, atlas cedarwood, lavender, and peppermint.

Romance

Aromatherapy can play a powerful role in relationships—in fact, some essential oils are so good at sparking passion that they're believed to be aphrodisiacs. Try inspiring feelings of love with sweet floral scents, spicing things up with citrus fragrances, or promoting connection with musky, earthy aromas.

STEAMY DIFFUSION

Put some love in the air with this blend of sweet ylang ylang and spicy cinnamon and ginger. (Ylang ylang also pairs well with citrus and clary sage.) Just drop these essential oils into an electric diffuser, adjusting the ratio as needed for your machine, and set it up in your bedroom.

Ylang Ylang
5 drops

Ginger
2 drops

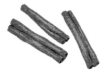

Cinnamon Bark
3 drops

SENSUAL MILK BATH

For a relaxing bath that you can enjoy together, combine cozy cardamom and the comforting yet romantic fragrances of rose and vanilla with 2 ounces (60 mL) coconut milk. Pour into a tub of warm water and use your hands to disperse the bath mixture.

Rose
3 drops

Cardamom
2 drops

Vanilla
2 drops

LOVE POTION MASSAGE OIL

Opt for opulence with this sensual massage blend, which will warm you up and get your blood flowing. Add these essential oils to 6 teaspoons carrier oil (such as grape-seed, coconut, or sweet almond), then take turns massaging each other's shoulders, neck, and back.

Sandalwood
6 drops

Vanilla
6 drops

Black Pepper
4 drops

LOVE-AT-FIRST-SCENT SACHETS

You can scent dried rosebuds with this pretty blend to create a passion-inspiring potpourri mix; just pour it into small cotton bags to make sachets, then store them in your lingerie drawer. (Or transfer the potpourri to a decorative bowl on your nightstand or dresser.)

Geranium
3 drops

Clary Sage
4 drops

Neroli
6 drops

ROMANTIC LINEN SPRAY

An intimate evening doesn't require heavy floral musks! You can set the scene with this more exotic aroma. Fill a 4-ounce (120-mL) spray bottle with ½ cup (120 mL) distilled water and these essential oils, then mist your linens.

Patchouli
45 drops

Vanilla
30 drops

Sandalwood
35 drops

Spruce
35 drops

ENCHANTRESS PERFUME

Try a bit of this evocative scent on the inside of your wrists, behind your ears, and on other pulse points. Drizzle the essential oils below into a 10-mL roll-on applicator, then fill the tube with a carrier oil of your choosing. Shake well before use.

Jasmine
4 drops

Frankincense
3 drops

Sweet Orange
3 drops

YLANG YLANG

One of my favorite floral scents, this essential oil comes
to us from the tropical yellow blossoms of the ylang
ylang plant. (If you're not sure how to pronounce
the name, it's *eee-lang eee-lang*. You might also see
it called ylang ylang extra or ylang ylang complete;
both make wonderful additions to your aromatherapy
toolkit.) This uplifting, stimulating oil enhances
feelings of gratitude and happiness, and its rich, exotic
scent is rumored to help a little romance bloom too.
Used topically, ylang ylang essential oil balances the
skin's oil production, making it a good choice for acne-
prone and oily skin. You'll also often spot it in scalp
treatments, as it's excellent at kick-starting hair growth.

| *Cananga odorata* | ORIGIN *Southeast Asia* |

Breezy Ylang Ylang + Rosehip Serum

1 tablespoon jojoba oil

1 tablespoon rosehip-seed oil

1 tablespoon rose water (see page 16)

5 drops ylang ylang essential oil

3 drops geranium essential oil

2-ounce (60-mL) spray bottle or roll-on applicator

Serums are personal—you need just the right weight and texture, plus hydration that doesn't make your skin feel greasy or cause breakouts. Rosehip-seed oil brims with vitamin C and omega-3, -6, and -9 fatty acids. It has amazing skin-rejuvenating benefits, and, when paired with ylang ylang essential oil, it makes a nourishing lotion that targets acne and wrinkles, as well as tones and brightens.

STEP 1 / Combine the jojoba oil, rosehip-seed oil, and rose water (learn how to make your own on page 16) in a small measuring cup with a spout. Stir to combine the ingredients.

STEP 2 / Drizzle the ylang ylang and geranium essential oils into your spray bottle or roll-on applicator.

STEP 3 / Carefully pour the oil mixture into the container with the essential oils. Screw on the lid and swirl gently to distribute the oils.

STEP 4 / To use, shake well and apply after cleansing or roll it on your skin throughout the day to alleviate dry skin. Use within 3 months.

Avocado Acne Mask

½ ripe avocado

1 tablespoon raw honey

1 drop ylang ylang essential oil

½ lemon

If you've battled acne, you're familiar with those annoying leftover red marks, known as post-inflammatory hyperpigmentation. They'll fade in time, but why not help hasten their departure with this mask? The avocado stimulates collagen production and cell regeneration, while the ylang ylang regulates oil. Don't forget the crucial lemon juice—it makes that hyperpigmentation a thing of the past.

STEP 1 / In a small bowl, mash the avocado until smooth.

STEP 2 / Add the honey and ylang ylang essential oil. Squeeze the half lemon over the mixture and stir until combined. (If you have sensitive skin, use less lemon or skip it altogether.)

STEP 3 / Wash your face and hands, then apply the mask and let it do its magic for 15 to 20 minutes. Wash off with warm water and follow with toner and moisturizer.

TIP / You can also apply it as a spot treatment for acne flare-ups or scars.

Healing Honey Hand Balm

¼ cup (50 g) coconut oil

¼ cup (60 mL) almond oil

¼ cup (60 mL) olive oil

5 tablespoons beeswax pellets

1 tablespoon shea butter

1½ tablespoons raw honey

36 drops ylang ylang essential oil

20 drops lemon essential oil

20 drops sandalwood essential oil

10-ounce (295-mL) glass jar

This homemade honey balm is the perfect antidote to all your dry-skin woes. While it makes an amazing hand salve, you can also use it as a cuticle cream, hair conditioner, or after-shower body lotion. But the real beauty of this balm is its honey, which locks in moisture and reduces dryness—even after you wash it off. I've also added floral ylang ylang, clean lemon, and woodsy sandalwood essential oils for a well-rounded scent that both stimulates and balances.

STEP 1 / Heat 2 inches (5 cm) of water in a small saucepan until it reaches a boil. Turn the heat to low.

STEP 2 / Combine the coconut, almond, and olive oils in a heat-safe glass bowl, then add the beeswax and shea butter.

STEP 3 / Place the glass bowl over the saucepan and heat until the oils and beeswax have completely melted. (You can also use a double boiler if you have one.)

STEP 4 / Remove the bowl from the heat and let the mixture cool slightly, then whisk in the honey. I recommend using raw honey for maximum skin-healing benefits. It delivers key amino acids, vitamins, enzymes, and antioxidants to skin cells, helping to nourish the skin and prevent free-radical damage.

STEP 5 / Drizzle in the ylang ylang, lemon, and sandalwood essential oils, then immediately pour the mixture into your glass jar. (Several small tins with lids would also work for a more portable option.)

STEP 6 / Let the balm cool to room temperature before use. Slather on a little bit every morning and you can wave goodbye to dry, cracked, irritated hands.

TIP / If you'd like a slightly different texture, remelt and re-create the balm with one of these changes: To make it firmer, add more beeswax; for a creamier, more spreadable option, add more of any of the three oils.

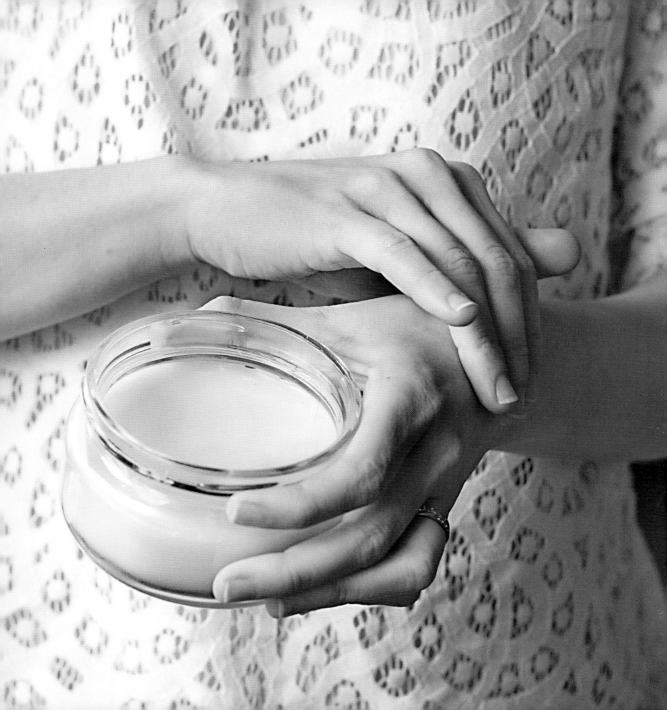

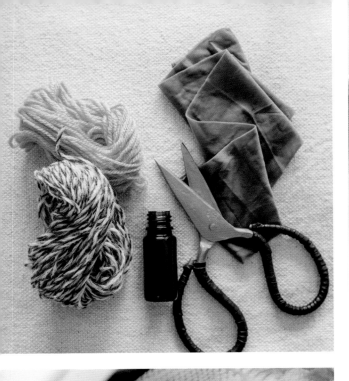

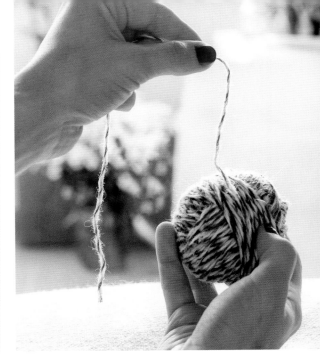

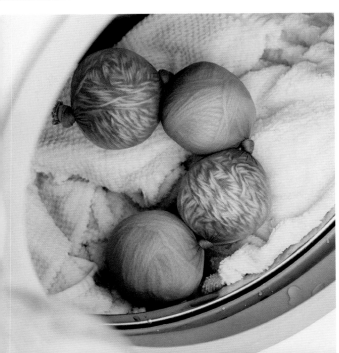

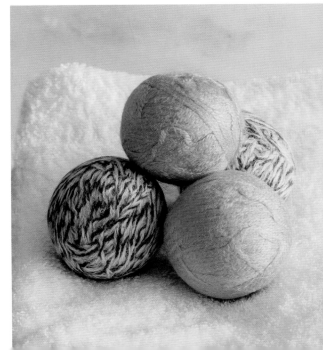

Heavenly Scented Dryer Balls

2 to 3 skeins scrap wool yarn (or even yarn from an old wool sweater)

Old pantyhose or tights

2 drops ylang ylang essential oil per yarn ball

Lots of nasty chemicals and fake fragrances get packed into seemingly harmless laundry helpers, and they all end up on your skin. These DIY wool dryer balls speed drying time, soften fabrics, and nix wrinkles without all those additives. For freshness, just add a few drops of ylang ylang essential oil before each use.

STEP 1 / Start by wrapping some wool yarn around two fingers about 10 times. (The exact amount needed will depend on the wool's thickness.)

STEP 2 / Remove the yarn from your fingers, then wrap it the opposite way until it's the size of a tennis ball.

STEP 3 / Place the yarn balls in the pantyhose or tights one by one, knotting the hose between each ball.

STEP 4 / Include the pantyhose-wrapped yarn balls in a few loads of laundry. Make sure the water is hot or they won't felt properly. Remove the balls from the pantyhose.

STEP 5 / Scent each ball with 2 drops ylang ylang essential oil, then pop them in with a wet dryer load. If they lose their effectiveness, send them back through the wash cycle and refresh the essential oil.

Homemade Fabric Softener Crystals

4 cups (1 kg) kosher salt

20 drops ylang ylang essential oil

24-ounce (710-mL) container

If your home has hard water, you know that the scratchy-towel struggle is real. To soften laundry that comes out of the wash stiff and rough to the touch, skip the irritating chemicals in store-bought fabric softener and make this all-natural version. It takes just two ingredients: kosher salt and your favorite essential oil.

STEP 1 / Add the kosher salt to a large mixing bowl. (Whatever you do, avoid using Epsom salt if you have hard water, as it will add minerals and make the water even harder.)

STEP 2 / Stir in the ylang ylang essential oil, then transfer the mixture to your large container.

STEP 3 / To use, add the salt to your load in the washer. A big load in hard water might need ¼ cup (70 g), while a small load might require as little as 1 tablespoon.

TIP / Cycles differ with front-load washers, so use this salt softener with caution. An all-natural softener using scented vinegar might be best.

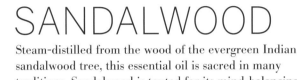

SANDALWOOD

Steam-distilled from the wood of the evergreen Indian sandalwood tree, this essential oil is sacred in many traditions. Sandalwood is touted for its mind-balancing powers and its protective effects on the epidermis, making it a mainstay in Ayurvedic therapies. Turn to it when dry, itchy skin needs soothing or when you need to extinguish an acne flare-up; or harness it as an aromatherapy tool to instill a sense of tranquility and inner peace. Sandalwood's strong earthy base note helps round out essential blends, so you'll often notice it wafting in fragrances and diffusions. It's helpful in times of stress or change because it fosters confidence, reduces irritability, and promotes emotional stability.

| *Santalum album* | ORIGIN *South Asia* |

Solid Sandalwood-Vanilla Perfume

1-ounce (30-mL) tin or tube
1 teaspoon almond oil
1½ teaspoons shea butter
1 teaspoon beeswax pellets
30 drops sandalwood essential oil prediluted in jojoba oil
20 drops vanilla essential oil prediluted in jojoba oil

If you're sensitive to fragrance, most perfumes are a no-go. But you can adjust this sweet and airy solid scent—providing both moisture and an uplifting aroma anytime, anywhere—to your own needs, no perfume headaches necessary.

STEP 1 / Select your container and place it nearby. Just about any small 1-ounce (30-mL) tin or jar will do, but chapstick tubes make the perfume especially easy to carry and apply.

STEP 2 / Add the almond oil, shea butter, and beeswax pellets to a heat-safe glass measuring cup.

STEP 3 / Pour 2 inches (5 cm) of water into a small saucepan. Place the measuring cup inside the

saucepan and bring the water to a simmer. Melt over medium heat.

STEP 4 / Remove the cup. Mix in the sandalwood and vanilla essential oils.

STEP 5 / Fill your tin or tube. Allow the mixture to harden completely before putting on the lid.

STEP 6 / Once it has cooled, toss it in your purse to use on the go. These lovelies will stay good for 6 months.

Anti-Aging Cucumber Eye Mask

½ cucumber, roughly chopped
2 tablespoons rose water (see page 16)
1 teaspoon evening primrose oil
2 drops sandalwood essential oil prediluted in jojoba oil
2 drops Roman chamomile essential oil
20 cotton face pads

With no oil glands to hydrate the delicate eye area, we need to step up our game to avoid pesky lines and crow's feet. This weekly mask with anti-inflammatory sandalwood and hydrating rose water helps de-puff, smooth, and tighten skin.

STEP 1 / In a blender, puree the cucumber and rose water until liquefied. (Refer to page 16 if making your own rose water.)

STEP 2 / Transfer to a bowl. Add the evening primrose oil and sandalwood and Roman chamomile essential oils.

STEP 3 / Soak the cotton pads in the mixture until thoroughly saturated, then squeeze out the excess.

STEP 4 / To use, place a pad under the eye close to the bottom lash line. Leave on for 10 to 15 minutes. Rinse and follow up with eye cream.

STEP 5 / Freeze the pads in a plastic zip-top bag for up to 1 year. Let them thaw for 10 minutes before use.

TIP / If you don't have cotton pads, soak a chamomile tea bag in the cucumber–rose water mixture instead.

Clay Medallion Diffuser

Package of terra cotta clay

Rolling pin

Circular lids or cookie cutters

Decorative stamps (optional)

Straw or toothpick

Twine

3 drops sandalwood essential oil
per medallion

2 drops bergamot essential oil
per medallion

Did you know terra cotta can absorb essential oils? That fun fact makes this porous clay perfect for scented crafts and gifts. You'll need to make indentations in the clay's surface so it can absorb the liquid oils, but no advanced art skills are required. Hang these decorative pieces at home or wherever you need an aromatherapy boost. The sandalwood essential oil will ground you, and it teams up nicely with the bergamot to melt away everyday worries.

STEP 1 / Warm a small chunk of clay in your hands to make it pliable.

STEP 2 / Use a rolling pin to press the clay into ⅛-inch (3-mm) to ¼-inch (6-mm) thickness.

STEP 3 / Trace around a circular lid with a knife. (You can also use cute cookie cutters, if you prefer.)

STEP 4 / Select pretty stamps and use them to press designs into the clay. Or try cutting slits in the clay with a knife—simple, clean graphics are your friend, if you're not particularly artistic.

STEP 5 / Use a straw or toothpick to make a hole in the top of the medallion that's large enough to accommodate your twine.

STEP 6 / Bake the clay following the package's directions. Remove it from the oven and let it cool completely.

STEP 7 / Thread your piece of twine through the hole and knot it. Drizzle the sandalwood and bergamot essential oils over the indentations and let them absorb into the clay.

STEP 8 / Repeat with the remaining medallions and then hang to enjoy their anxiety-reducing scent. You can also incorporate these into your presents as gift tags. If the fragrance starts to fade over time, simply add more drops of essential oil.

TIP / These also make great refrigerator magnets. Skip the hole and string—use a hot-glue gun to adhere a magnet to the back instead.

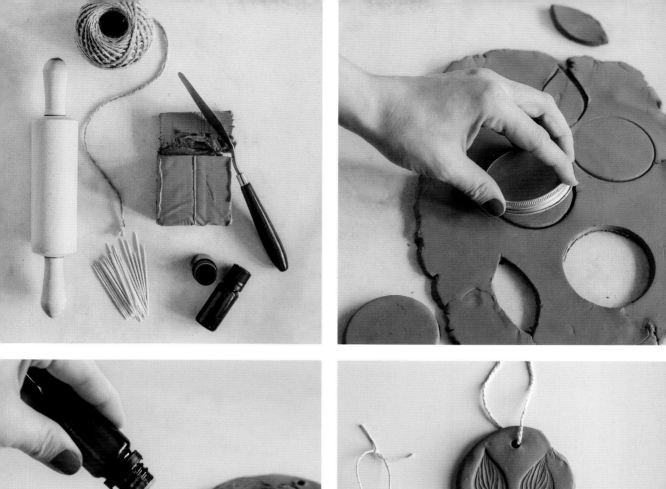

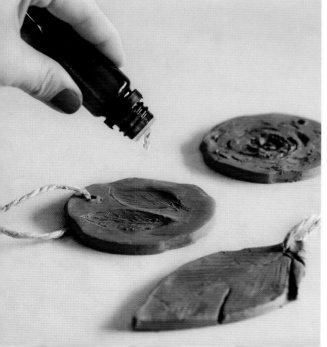

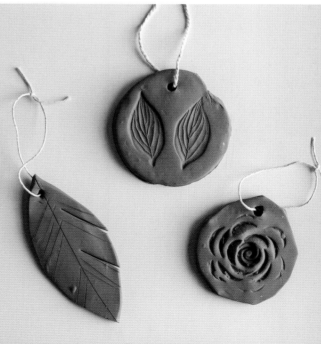

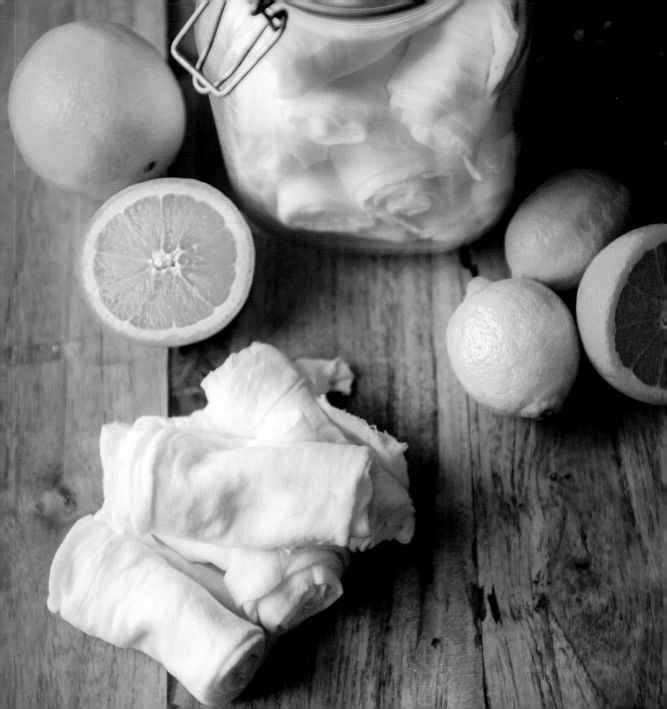

Are dirty floors and furniture your nemeses? With all the splatters, dust, crumbs, and foot- and paw prints of everyday life, my floor definitely requires regular maintenance. That's why it's important to use cleaners that do the job, come with the right price tag, and aren't full of potentially toxic chemicals. Try treating your wood floor and furniture with these simple recipes that combine the warm, earthy aroma of sandalwood and the fresh scent of citrus.

All-Surface Floor Cleaner

1 cup (240 mL) rubbing alcohol

1 cup (240 mL) distilled white vinegar

30 drops sandalwood essential oil prediluted in joboba oil

20 drops sweet orange essential oil

1 gallon (3.25 L) very hot tap water

Add the rubbing alcohol, distilled white vinegar, sandalwood and sweet orange essential oils, and water to a large bucket and attack your floors as needed. For tough jobs, reduce the water to 3 quarts (3 L) and add 1 teaspoon dish soap to cut grease.

Make-It-Gleam Furniture Polish

2 tablespoons beeswax

½ cup (120 mL) olive oil

24 drops sandalwood essential oil prediluted in joboba oil

1 teaspoon lemon essential oil

5-ounce (150-mL) lidded container

Combine the beeswax and olive oil in a spouted heat-safe glass measuring cup. Heat it in short bursts in the microwave, stirring frequently, until the beeswax has melted. Add the sandalwood and lemon essential oils, then pour the mixture into your container. To give the polish a smooth consistency, continue to stir until it's room temperature. Gently rub it into dull wood surfaces with a clean, lint-free dusting cloth.

Wood Furniture Wipes

2 tablespoons olive oil

20 drops sandalwood essential oil prediluted in jojoba oil

10 drops lemon essential oil

24-ounce (710-mL) spray bottle

1 tablespoon vinegar or lemon juice

3 cups (710 mL) distilled water

8 soft, lint-free cloths

24-ounce (710-mL) jar

Pour the olive oil and sandalwood and lemon essential oils into the spray bottle, then add the vinegar or lemon juice and the distilled water. Shake well and then spritz each cloth until damp. Roll the cloths and store in a jar with a tight-fitting lid. Use to dust within 3 months.

Hardwood Floor Cleaner

1 cup (240 mL) water

1 black tea bag

1 gallon (3.25 L) hot water

1 tablespoon olive oil

½ cup (120 mL) vinegar

15 drops sandalwood essential oil prediluted in joboba oil

Bring 1 cup (240 mL) of water to a boil and steep the black tea bag, allowing it to cool to room temperature. In the meantime, fill a bucket with 1 gallon (3.25 L) of hot water. Add the black tea, olive oil, vinegar, and sandalwood essential oil. Use it with a mop to clean your floors as usual; you'll see the tannic acid in the tea and olive oil restore shine. Dry-mop after cleaning if your floors are too slippery.

Uplift

CHAPTER TWO

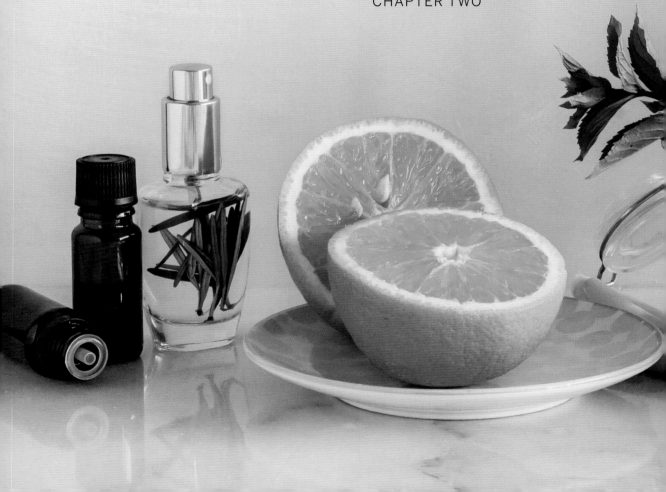

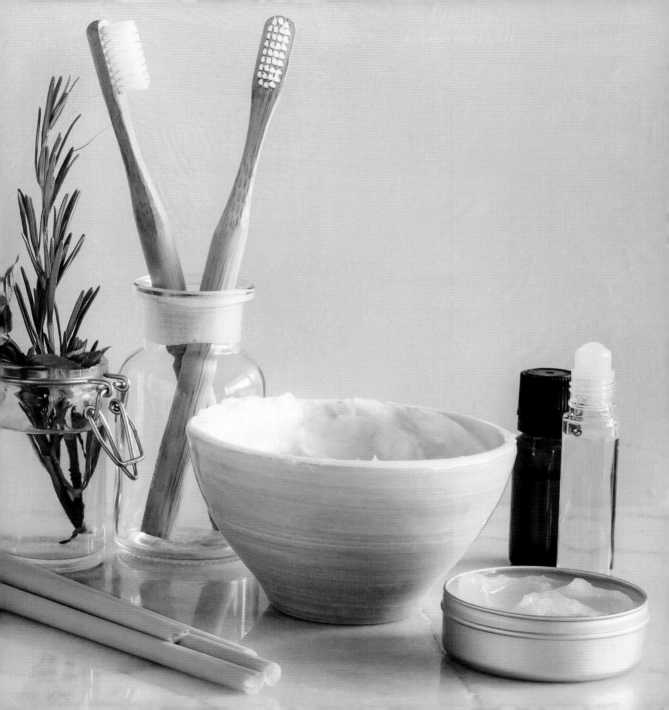

PEPPERMINT

Ah, peppermint. You know it as soon as you smell
that crisp, invigorating scent. Peppermint is one of
the most commonly used essential oils, with countless
applications for your health and home. Its menthol
content can help clear up the symptoms of congestion,
and it's a must for relieving tension when you're
overwhelmed or stuck staring at a computer. This
peppy plant is also antiseptic and antiviral, and its cool,
tingling sensation stimulates circulation and relaxes sore
muscles. Peppermint is great to call on in beauty too: It
makes an excellent astringent toner, and it commonly
cameos in treatments for oily and acne-prone skin.

| *Mentha piperita* | ORIGIN *Europe* |

Sweet Dreams Mattress Detox Mix

½ cup (110 g) baking soda

12 drops peppermint
essential oil

10 drops eucalyptus
essential oil

10 drops tea tree
essential oil

5 drops clove bud essential oil

4-ounce (120-mL) container
with a shaker top

Your body needs rest to detox, so it's important to hit the hay in a healthy bed that promotes a good night's sleep—which means ridding your linens of allergens and dust mites. A simple combination of baking soda and essential oils will deodorize, eliminate moisture, and kill unwelcome parasites in your mattress.

STEP 1 / Dump the baking soda into a small bowl. Add the peppermint, eucalyptus, tea tree, and clove bud essential oils. Stir together.

STEP 2 / Pour the mixture into a container with a shaker top. (Or you can poke holes in the lid of a jar or put an old spice bottle to new use.)

STEP 3 / Strip the linens off the bed and wash them in hot water with a few drops of eucalyptus essential oil. Then sprinkle the entire baking soda mixture onto the bare mattress; let it sit for at least 1 hour and up to 48 hours—the longer the better.

STEP 4 / Vacuum up the mixture and replace the linens when dry.

Peppermint Pump Hand Soap

1 cup (240 mL) peppermint
hydrosol (see page 16)

1 cup (240 mL) liquid
castile soap

2 tablespoons sweet almond oil

25 drops peppermint
essential oil

16-ounce (475-mL) pump
bottle

Whipping up your own hand soap is a game changer. It is simple to make, saves money, and cheers me up every time I wash my hands with its fresh, revitalizing peppermint scent. This essential oil is great for irritated skin, and, when paired with peppermint hydrosol, it really refreshes hardworking hands.

STEP 1 / Make the peppermint hydrosol following the instructions on page 16.

STEP 2 / Measure and add the unscented liquid castile soap, sweet almond oil, and peppermint essential oil to the hydrosol, then stir.

STEP 3 / Pour the mixture into your pump bottle. To use, dispense 1 to 2 pumps of soap into your hands and lather.

TIP / To modify this recipe into a surprisingly heavy-duty dish soap, add 1½ teaspoons super washing soda to the peppermint hydrosol. Add the unscented liquid castile soap, peppermint essential oil, and 1 tablespoon sweet almond oil. Stir the mixture to dissolve, then add 1 to 2 teaspoons to a sink of hot water and see your dishes sparkle.

Minty-Fresh Coconut Toothpaste

3 tablespoons coconut oil

3-ounce (90-mL) container

3 tablespoons baking soda

10 drops peppermint
essential oil

Once you try homemade toothpaste, you'll never go back. The common cleansing ingredient in most store-bought stuff—sodium lauryl sulfate—can cause mouth sores and inflammation. This naturally antiseptic and antiviral DIY version offers the same cleansing action without all that irritation—plus, its peppermint essential oil helps boost gum health and makes your breath minty fresh.

STEP 1 / If your coconut oil is solid, stick it in the microwave for a few seconds. No need to liquefy—just warm and soften it so you can blend it with the other ingredients.

STEP 2 / Transfer the coconut oil to your container, then stir in the baking soda and peppermint essential oil.

STEP 3 / Apply to your toothbrush and brush your teeth as normal. (You might have to spit and reapply the toothpaste after 45 seconds or so, as the mixture turns to liquid fast.) Use within 1 month.

TIP / If you don't like the bracing peppermint taste, add a bit of stevia to sweeten things up.

Skin-Quenching Sunburn Spray

1 cup (240 mL) distilled water

2 peppermint tea bags

1 green tea bag

1 chamomile tea bag

8-ounce (240-mL) spray bottle

¼ cup (60 mL) aloe vera gel

1 tablespoon vegetable glycerin
(or fractionated coconut oil)

1 tablespoon apple cider vinegar

12 drops peppermint
essential oil

10 drops lavender essential oil

The flip side of a day at the beach is a day—or three—of itching and peeling. Despite diligently wearing sunscreen and hats, the sun occasionally gets the better of us. With its cooling peppermint tea, this spray takes the sting out of sunburns and helps prevent peeling. Try it just out of the fridge for instant relief.

STEP 1 / Bring the distilled water to a boil in a saucepan; remove from the heat. Add the peppermint, green, and chamomile tea bags. Steep for about 10 minutes, then discard the used bags. Let the tea cool completely.

STEP 2 / Pour ½ cup (120 mL) of the tea into your spray bottle. (You can reserve the rest of the tea in the fridge for up to 2 weeks.)

STEP 3 / Add the aloe vera gel, vegetable glycerin or fractionated coconut oil, apple cider vinegar, and peppermint and lavender essential oils to the spray bottle. Swirl to combine the ingredients.

STEP 4 / Shake before each use, then spritz anywhere your skin is red and irritated. Follow with plenty of moisturizer. Store in the refrigerator and use within 2 weeks.

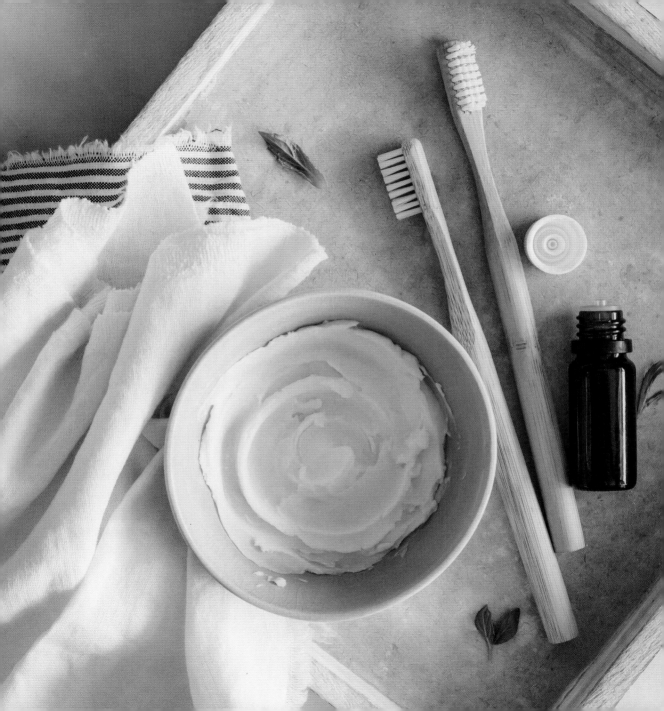

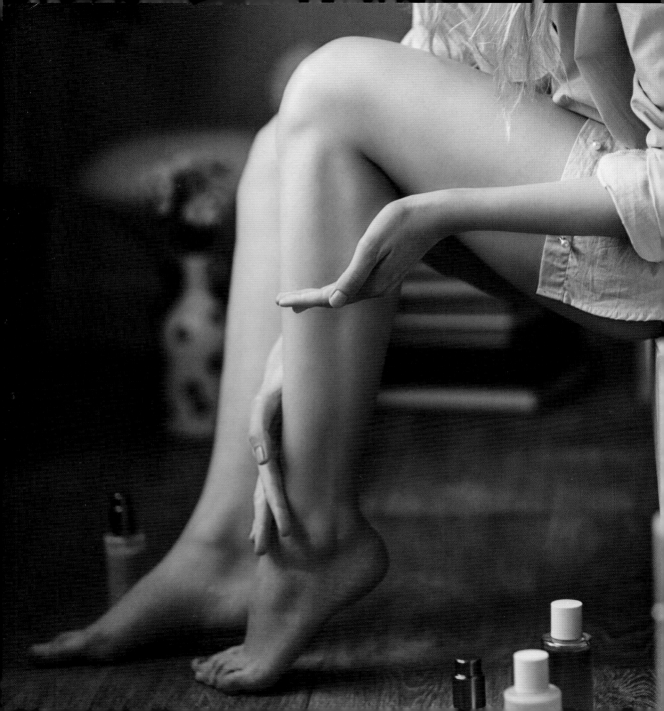

Our feet need extra exfoliation to slough off the dead skin that collects on our heels, along with extra moisture to prevent painful cracking. These at-home treatments provide all that and more for adventure-weary soles. The cooling action of peppermint relieves achy feet and combats odor—plus, the scent is mood-lifting. So grab a basin, a towel, and these ingredients to give your feet some much-needed nurturing.

Citrus-Mint Foot Soak

½ cup (120 g) Epsom salt

1 orange, sliced

8 cups (475 mL) warm water

6 drops peppermint essential oil

2 teaspoons carrier oil, such as jojoba or sweet almond

Put the Epsom salt and orange slices in a large basin and pour in the warm water. Dilute the peppermint essential oil with your carrier oil and swirl it in the water. Soak your feet in the mixture for a good 20 minutes, then towel-dry and moisturize.

Refreshing Foot Scrub

2 tablespoons sugar

1 teaspoon lemon juice

2 teaspoons honey

1 tablespoon olive oil

6 drops peppermint essential oil

Combine the sugar, lemon juice, honey, olive oil, and peppermint essential oil in a bowl. Gently scrub the mixture onto your feet, especially your heels and any calloused areas. Soak two hand towels in hot water, wring them out, and cover your feet for 5 minutes before wiping off the scrub. Rinse under warm water.

Moisture-Lock Massage Oil

¼ cup (60 mL) sweet almond oil

2-ounce (60-mL) bottle

12 drops peppermint essential oil

10 drops tea tree essential oil

Pour the sweet almond oil into your bottle. Drizzle in the peppermint and tea tree essential oils, then recap the bottle and swirl to blend. Apply to your feet after a soak and scrub, massaging it into your soles and toes for a moisturizing treat. Use within 6 months.

Odor-Banishing Shoe Powder

¼ cup (50 g) baking soda

¼ cup (30 g) cornstarch

20 drops peppermint essential oil

4-ounce (120-mL) jar

Combine the baking soda and cornstarch in a small bowl. Add the peppermint essential oil and stir, breaking up any clumps, and then transfer to the jar. To use, rub 1 teaspoon into your soles and sprinkle a dash inside your shoes before slipping them on—it'll absorb any and all odors. Use within 1 year.

SWEET ORANGE

You know that freshly peeled orange scent—intoxicating and bright, it immediately perks you up and chases blues away. Typically referred to as sweet orange, this essential oil gets its uplifting aroma from the compound limonene, which also provides it with the impressive antiseptic properties that make it a mainstay in cleaning products for both home and body. Used topically, sweet orange essential oil improves collagen production and stimulates circulation and toxin removal. Plus, this essential oil is easily captured from the fruit peel, making it an affordable addition to your collection—so keep this perky and powerful elixir in heavy rotation!

| *Citrus sinensis* | ORIGIN *Southern China* |

Cleaning the bathroom is enough of a pain, but factor in the chemical smells of store-bought disinfectants (plus the eco-guilt that comes with using them) and it's enough to make you put off that chore indefinitely. Sweet orange essential oil's antibacterial properties make it a great addition to homemade cleaners—just add liquid castile soap, distilled water, baking soda, and vinegar, and you'll have an arsenal of all-natural products that can take on even the grossest room in the house.

Antibacterial Foaming Handwash

2 tablespoons unscented liquid castile soap

12 drops sweet orange essential oil

10-ounce (295-mL) pump bottle

10 ounces (295 mL) distilled water

Add the unscented liquid castile soap and sweet orange essential oil to your pump dispenser. Fill the bottle to the top with distilled water and swirl to combine. Replace the lid and foam up! Use within 3 months.

Homemade Soft Scrub

½ cup (110 g) baking soda

2 tablespoons liquid castile soap

8 drops sweet orange essential oil

4 drops tea tree essential oil

Mix the baking soda and liquid castile soap in a bowl. Stir until combined, then drizzle in the sweet orange and tea tree essential oils. Use a sponge to scrub the mixture all over sinks and tubs (or pretty much any surface in the bathroom). Rinse well afterward.

See-Glass-Sparkle Cleaning Spray

10 drops sweet orange essential oil

16-ounce (475-mL) spray bottle

2 tablespoons rubbing alcohol

2 tablespoons distilled white vinegar

1 tablespoon cornstarch

1½ cups (355 mL) distilled water

Drizzle the sweet orange essential oil into your spray bottle, then pour in the rubbing alcohol and distilled white vinegar. Swirl the bottle to disperse the essential oil. Add the cornstarch and distilled water, then replace bottle's top. Shake well and spritz onto windows or any other glass surface, then wipe down with a sheet of newspaper or a terry-cloth towel.

All-Mighty Toilet Volcano

2 tablespoons unscented liquid castile soap

½ cup (120 mL) distilled white vinegar

15 drops sweet orange essential oil

½ cup (110 g) baking soda

Pour the unscented liquid castile soap, distilled white vinegar, and sweet orange essential oil straight into the toilet bowl. Let it sit for 10 minutes, then dump in the baking soda. (Important: If you pour it in too early, you'll get club soda—not the powerhouse cleaner you were hoping for.) Wait for the bubbles to die down, then scrub the toilet and flush.

So Zen Yoga Mat Mist

1 ounce (30 mL) vodka or witch hazel

2-ounce (60-mL) spray bottle

20 drops sweet orange essential oil

6 drops lavender essential oil

1 ounce (30 mL) orange blossom water or distilled water

Catch a whiff of something unpleasant during downward dog? After a few intense yoga sessions, your trusty mat may be in need of a refresh—but you can skip those silly and pricey yoga mat spray products. This simple homemade mist will not only kill stink-causing bacteria, it will leave a calming citrus-floral scent that promotes mental clarity. Now that's something to om about.

STEP 1 / Pour the alcohol into your spray bottle. Drizzle in the sweet orange and lavender essential oils.

STEP 2 / Replace the bottle cap and swirl to combine the ingredients. Let the essential oils dissolve in the alcohol for 20 minutes.

STEP 3 / Pour in the orange blossom water or distilled water and replace the cap. Shake again.

STEP 4 / To use, first agitate the bottle, then spritz it over your yoga mat. Wipe down the mat immediately with a towel. Use within 3 months.

Luscious Coconut-Citrus Soap

2 pounds (910 g) melt-and-pour shea butter soap base

¼ cup (20 g) shredded coconut

2 tablespoons orange zest

1 tablespoon sweet orange essential oil

What can you make with orange, coconut, and a cake pan? Sure, you could whip up a delicious dessert, but this recipe results in a homemade soap that smells heavenly—and is a piece of cake to make too. The sunny orange scent will improve your mood while the shea and coconut soothe hardworking hands.

STEP 1 / Cut your shea butter soap base into chunks and add them to a heat-safe glass bowl.

STEP 2 / Microwave the soap in 30-second increments until it's completely melted, then stir in the shredded coconut and orange zest.

STEP 3 / Stir the mixture until well combined. When it's cool enough that a thin layer develops on the surface, stir in the sweet orange essential oil.

STEP 4 / Pour the mixture into a nonstick cake pan and let it sit for 2 to 3 hours. When firm, turn the soap out of the pan onto a cutting board and cut it into bars of your desired size. Let the soap sit for 3 days before sudsing up with one. Use within 6 months.

TIP / Lining the nonstick cake pan with wax paper will make it easier to remove the soap. It'll also keep the soap's bottom nice and smooth.

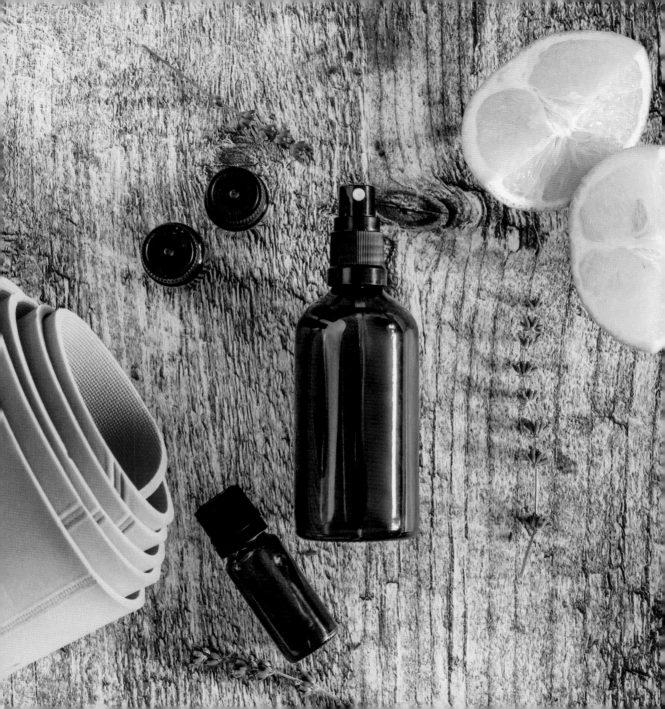

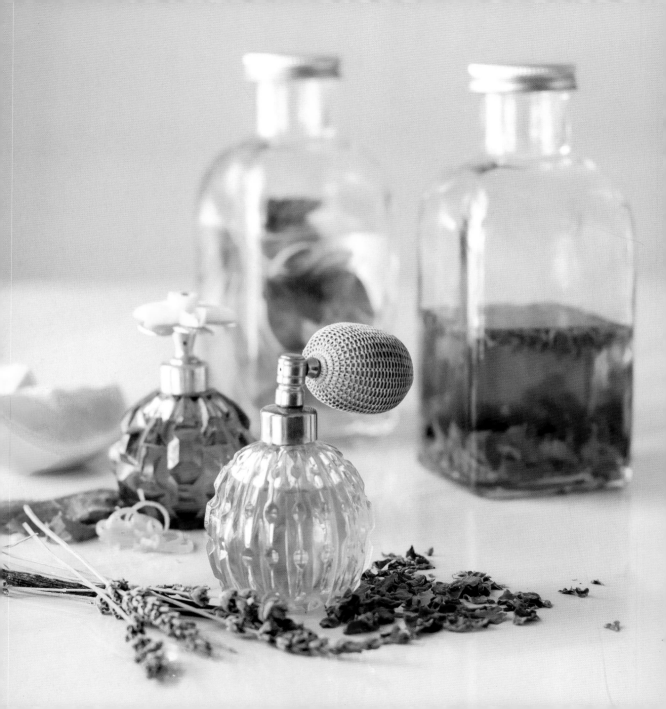

Have-It-Your-Way Personalized Perfume

Peel from 1 orange

¼ cup (6 g) fresh mint leaves

8-ounce (240-mL) glass jar

1 cup (240 mL) vodka

1 tablespoon jojoba oil

2-ounce (60-mL) dark
glass container

10 drops grapefruit essential oil

12 drops sweet orange
essential oil

5 drops peppermint essential oil

5 drops lavender essential oil

1 tablespoon distilled water

Pretty perfume bottle (optional)

Finding a perfume you like—and that you can afford—is no easy task. But this DIY version is an inexpensive, customizable way to get exactly the fragrance that suits you. Clean citrus scents, such as sweet orange, not only smell divine—they can energize and boost creativity, lifting brain fog and helping you hit refresh. For additional subtle scent, I infuse the booze with fresh ingredients.

STEP 1 / To infuse the vodka, put the orange peel and mint leaves in your clean, dry jar. Pour in the vodka and replace the lid, then shake the jar to fully submerse the citrus and mint.

STEP 2 / Let the jar sit for at least 2 weeks (4 to 6 is even better), shaking the jar occasionally. Strain and discard the peel and mint.

STEP 3 / Pour the jojoba oil into your container, then add 2 tablespoons of the infused alcohol. (Keep the infused booze for your next perfume batch—or mix up a cocktail!)

STEP 4 / Drizzle in the grapefruit essential oil (your base note), followed by the sweet orange and peppermint essential oils (your middle notes). Finish with the lavender essential oil as your top note.

STEP 5 / Let the essential oils diffuse into the mixture for at least 20 minutes. Add the distilled water, replace the cap, and swirl to mix.

STEP 6 / Store for at least 48 hours or up to 6 weeks—the longer it sits, the stronger the aroma. Transfer the liquid to a pretty perfume bottle once it reaches your desired intensity.

STEP 7 / Apply it to pulse points, like the insides of your wrists and behind your ears. Use within 6 months.

BUILDING FRAGRANCES 101

A well-balanced perfume includes top, middle, and base notes. We tend to notice top notes first, but their scents dissipate the fastest. Middle and base notes add staying power as well as fullness and depth. Here are where a few favorite essential oils fall in the scent categories.

TOP NOTES Anise, sweet basil, bergamot, eucalyptus, grapefruit, lavender, lemon, lemongrass, lime, mandarin, peppermint, spearmint, sweet orange, and tangerine.
MIDDLE NOTES Black pepper, cinnamon leaf, clary sage, clove bud, cypress, fennel, geranium,

juniper, neroli, nutmeg, palmarosa, pine, Roman chamomile, rose, rosemary, spruce, thyme, and ylang ylang.
BASE NOTES Atlas cedarwood, frankincense, ginger, helichrysum, myrrh, patchouli, sandalwood, vanilla, and vetiver.

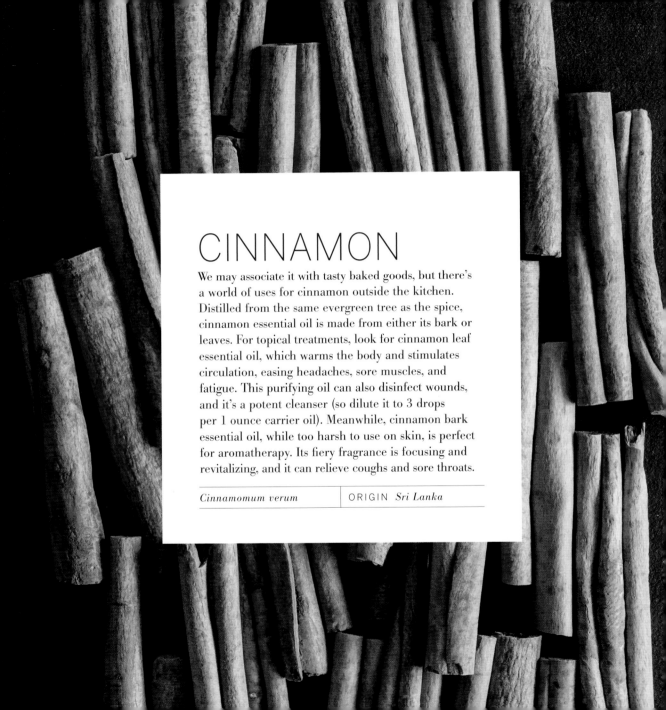

CINNAMON

We may associate it with tasty baked goods, but there's a world of uses for cinnamon outside the kitchen. Distilled from the same evergreen tree as the spice, cinnamon essential oil is made from either its bark or leaves. For topical treatments, look for cinnamon leaf essential oil, which warms the body and stimulates circulation, easing headaches, sore muscles, and fatigue. This purifying oil can also disinfect wounds, and it's a potent cleanser (so dilute it to 3 drops per 1 ounce carrier oil). Meanwhile, cinnamon bark essential oil, while too harsh to use on skin, is perfect for aromatherapy. Its fiery fragrance is focusing and revitalizing, and it can relieve coughs and sore throats.

| *Cinnamomum verum* | ORIGIN *Sri Lanka* |

Warming Massage Candles

3 ounces (85 g) soy wax flakes

4-ounce (120-mL) heat-safe glass jar

Candlewick

2 wooden craft sticks

2 tablespoons grape-seed oil

½ teaspoon vitamin E oil (or 2 capsules)

10 drops sandalwood essential oil

6 drops patchouli essential oil

4 drops cinnamon leaf essential oil

4 drops sweet orange essential oil

No time (or cash) for a proper massage? A cinnamon massage candle is the next best thing: It melts easily, you can pour the wax right onto your skin, and the warm, familiar scent boosts self-confidence and increases feelings of security. Cinnamon leaf oil can also relieve muscles and joints when applied topically. Because it's so potent, use it in small doses and dilute it well.

STEP 1 / Measure the soy wax flakes and heat them in a spouted heat-safe glass measuring cup until completely melted (approximately 90 seconds).

STEP 2 / Clean and dry your jar. (You can also try sourcing a cute dish, such as a creamer pitcher, teacup, or gravy boat, from a thrift store.) Place the wick in the jar so that it stands up straight with the tab pressed to the bottom. Help keep the wick in place by laying a wooden craft stick across the jar on each side of the wick.

STEP 3 / Add the grape-seed oil to the melted wax and stir together. Then drizzle in the vitamin E oil and the sandalwood, patchouli, cinnamon leaf, and sweet orange essential oils, and stir again.

STEP 4 / Carefully pour the mixture into the jar and let it set for about 1 hour. Once the candle wax solidifies, trim the wick to ¼ inch (6 mm).

STEP 5 / To use, light the candle and let it burn for 15 to 20 minutes, allowing a small pool of wax to form around the wick. Blow it out and then carefully pour some of the wax into your hand, or dip the tips of your fingers into the wax and massage the oil into the skin.

STEP 6 / After the massage, cover the candle to prevent dust particles from settling on the surface. Allow the wax to reharden and use again and again within 6 months.

TIP / While massage candles are totally safe to use on the skin, it's a good idea to test a small amount of the warm oil on the inside of your wrist before trying it elsewhere, just to make sure it won't irritate your skin. Avoid using the oil on the face or other sensitive areas, and always practice fire safety when burning your candle.

Lip-Plumping Cinnamon Balm

1½ tablespoons beeswax pellets

4 tablespoons sweet almond oil

½ teaspoon vitamin E oil
(or 2 capsules)

¾ tablespoon honey

4 drops cinnamon leaf
essential oil

6 ½-ounce (15-mL) lip balm
containers

When the weather cools and it seems like all moisture has been sucked from the air, dry and chapped lips are inevitable. This homemade balm comes to your rescue with vitamin E oil to hydrate and cinnamon leaf essential oil to warm skin and boost circulation, which naturally "plumps" your lips—no collagen required!

STEP 1 / Mix the beeswax pellets and sweet almond oil in a spouted heat-safe glass measuring cup.

STEP 2 / Pour 2 inches (5 cm) of water into a small saucepan and heat it on low. Place the measuring cup in the water to melt the wax and oil together. (You can also use a double boiler if you have one.)

STEP 3 / Remove the glass from the water. Pour in the vitamin E oil, then add the honey and cinnamon leaf essential oil. Stir to combine.

STEP 4 / Carefully pour the mixture into your six lip balm containers. (Work fast because the beeswax will harden quickly!) Make sure to use within 6 months.

Sugar + Spice Body Scrub

1 cup (200 g) sugar

¼ cup (50 g) brown sugar

1 tablespoon ground cinnamon

1 teaspoon vanilla extract

6 drops cinnamon leaf
essential oil

½ cup (120 mL) grape-seed oil

16-ounce (475-mL) container

Forget cookies—this fragrant scrub will fill your house with the scents of cinnamon and vanilla. Rich in antioxidants, it uses cinnamon essential oil to warm the body, stimulate circulation, and fight off the winter blahs. Vanilla extract adds a touch of sweetness that entices and calms.

STEP 1 / Combine the granulated and brown sugars with the ground cinnamon in a small bowl. Mix thoroughly.

STEP 2 / Add the vanilla extract and cinnamon leaf essential oil. Remember, this oil is potent, so easy does it.

STEP 3 / Slowly add in the grape-seed oil. Depending on your desired consistency, add more oil

(to make it looser and more moisturizing) or more sugar, which will create a thicker mixture that's easier to scoop.

STEP 4 / Transfer the scrub to a container and add the lid. To use, scoop out a handful and massage in small circles on damp skin, focusing on rough areas like the elbows and knees, before rinsing off. Use within 6 weeks.

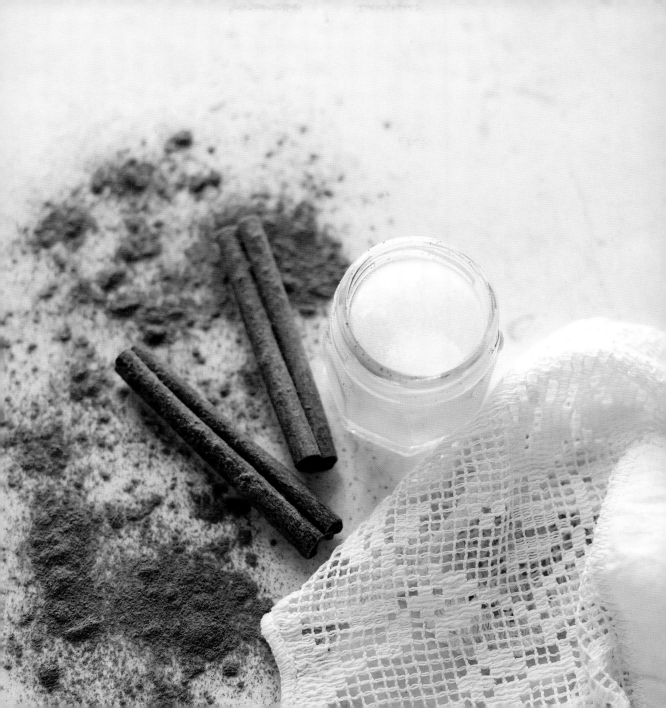

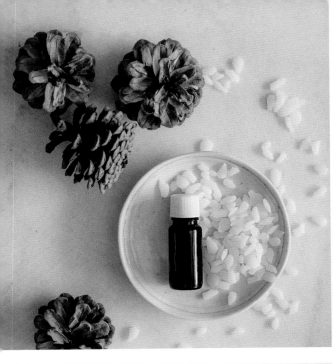
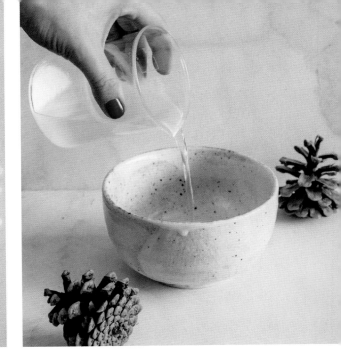
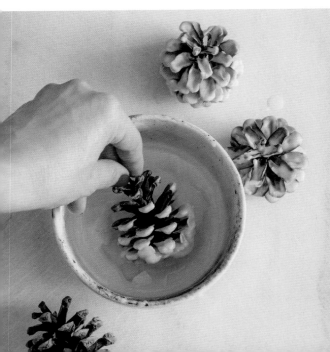
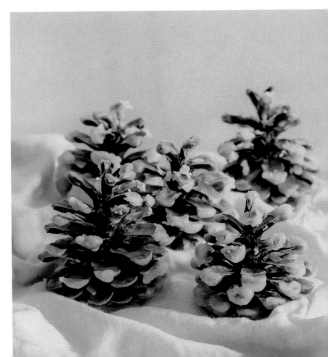

Scented Pinecone Fire Starters

1 cup (90 g) soy wax flakes

15 drops cinnamon bark essential oil

10 to 12 pinecones

It's easy to go overboard with holiday crafts—all those Pinterest-worthy cookies and fussy handmade ornaments! This year, try these easy wax-dipped pinecone firestarters instead. They're pretty enough to gift, and their cinnamon scent will make you want to spend the whole season cozying up in front of the fireplace.

STEP 1 / Add the soy wax flakes to a heat-safe glass bowl. Heat in 30-second blasts, stirring in between each, until the wax fully melts.

STEP 2 / Drizzle in the cinnamon bark essential oil and stir, then dip the pinecones into the wax mixture (no need to cover them completely) and set them on wax paper to dry.

STEP 3 / Continue dipping and drying each pinecone several times to build up a thick coat of wax.

STEP 4 / After the pinecones dry, you may choose to keep them as decor—freshening the scent with a few drops of essential oil as needed—or to use in the fireplace. Just toss them in and get a good blaze going.

Cold-Busting Pot Simmer

20 drops clove bud essential oil

18 drops lemon essential oil

10 drops cinnamon bark essential oil

8 drops eucalyptus essential oil

5 drops rosemary essential oil

5-mL amber bottle

4 cups (945 mL) water

A pot simmer is a great way to make your home smell amazing—and it can help strengthen your respiratory system and relieve coughs. This blend combines five essential oils with antiseptic, antiviral, and antimicrobial powers to purify the air; plus, it scents the room with the comforting aromas of clove bud and cinnamon.

STEP 1 / Drizzle the clove bud, lemon, cinnamon bark, eucalyptus, and rosemary essential oils into your amber bottle. Replace the lid and swirl the bottle to mix the oils.

STEP 2 / Fill a small saucepan with the water and heat on low. Pour in 5 drops of the blend and let simmer for 30 minutes, adding water as needed to keep the good aromas flowing through your home. Repeat up to 4 times a day, as needed.

TIP / Note that this recipe shouldn't be used around children under 10. If you're pregnant or breastfeeding, replace the cinnamon bark with cinnamon leaf essential oil.

Air Freshness

Take it from someone who knows: Exploring ways to scent your home is one of the fastest ways to get hooked on essential oils. Diffusing them not only affects our moods, it also purifies the air around us. Whether you're deep-cleaning or relaxing by a fire, these simple blends will make you want to breathe deep.

CLEAN-SLATE POT SIMMER

Just cooked dinner and now your whole kitchen smells a little fishy? Fill a saucepan with water, add these essential oils, and heat over low for between 15 and 20 minutes.

SECRET WEAPON BATHROOM MIST

Keep this spray handy in the bathroom to mask tough odors. Combine the following essential oils in 4 ounces (120 mL) water for a scent that you actually want to smell!

QUICK PRE-COMPANY CARPET DEODORIZER

Next time you need your space to smell great in a hurry, add these essential oils to 1 cup (220 g) baking soda. Sprinkle the whole box over the carpet, let it sit for 30 minutes, and vacuum up the evidence.

Lime
4 drops

Clove Bud
2 drops

Atlas Cedarwood
60 drops

Lemon
60 drops

Patchouli
10 drops

Vetiver
10 drops

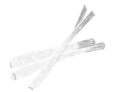
Lemongrass
2 drops

Clove Bud
30 drops

Lime
20 drops

COZY AROMATIC FIREWOOD CHIPS

On the next brrr-inducingly cold day, bring the outdoors in with scented firewood chips. Add the following essential oils to 1 pound (455 g) dry hardwood chips, then toss a few on the fire to enjoy their woodsy scent.

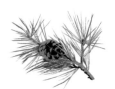

Pine
18 drops

Spruce
18 drops

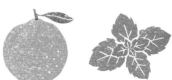

Sweet Orange
18 drops

Peppermint
9 drops

FINE-FALL-DAY POTPOURRI MIX

Scented dried orange slices make a simple potpourri for crisp autumn weather. Combine the dried oranges with these spicy essential oils in a small decorative bowl. Refresh the scent to keep the season going.

Nutmeg
2 drops

Clove Bud
1 drop

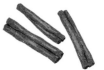

Cinnamon Bark
2 drops

SIMPLE SCENTED SALT DIFFUSER

A salt diffuser is one of the easiest ways to purify the air and send your own custom scent wafting through the air. Mix these essential oils with 1 cup (290 g) sea salt in a shallow bowl or candle holder, then nestle an unscented candle in the center of the dish to release this warm scent.

Sweet Orange
10 drops

Patchouli
6 drops

Vanilla
4 drops

Cinnamon Bark
2 drops

ATLAS CEDARWOOD

This warm, timbery scent has long been an aromatic pillar; it goes all the way back to Egyptian embalming rituals. The stabilizing essential oil is steam-distilled from the wood of the hardy Atlas cedarwood trees of Algeria and Morocco, which symbolize wisdom and majesty. (Steer clear of non-Atlas cedarwood oils, including Virginian—it's sourced from juniper trees.) As an antiseptic, this essential oil comes to the rescue if you're battling acne or eczema, and it also works as an astringent to tone oily skin and cleanse hair. As a final bonus, it deters pests such as moths and mosquitoes.

| *Cedrus atlantica* | ORIGIN *Northern Africa* |

Itch-Easing Eczema Salve

1 tablespoon calendula-infused oil (see page 16)

2 tablespoons shea butter

2 teaspoons beeswax pellets

10 drops Atlas cedarwood essential oil

6 drops geranium essential oil

6 drops lavender essential oil

2-ounce (60-mL) glass jar

Inflammation, dryness, rash—all describe eczema, a common skin condition that tends to flare up at the worst possible times. Since there isn't a cure, it's all about managing symptoms and triggers, and this balm will do the trick. Shea butter is a rich moisturizer and a source of skin-healing vitamin A, while Atlas cedarwood essential oil contributes anti-inflammatory compounds that relieve itchy skin.

STEP 1 / For an antioxidant-rich, skin-repairing boost, make a calendula-infused oil using the instructions on page 16.

STEP 2 / Pour 2 inches (5 cm) of water into a saucepan and bring to a boil. Lower the heat, then combine the infused oil, shea butter, and beeswax in a heat-safe glass bowl. Place the bowl over the saucepan.

STEP 3 / Once the mixture has melted, remove the bowl from heat. Add the Atlas cedarwood, geranium, and lavender essential oils.

STEP 4 / Transfer the mixture to the jar and let it sit until completely cool.

STEP 5 / For relief, apply a thin layer to affected areas as often as needed. Use within 6 months.

Calming Colloidal Oatmeal Bath

1 cup (90 g) old-fashioned oats

½ cup (110 g) baking soda

1 tablespoon grape-seed oil

6 drops Atlas cedarwood essential oil

Nothing tames the maddening itch of poison ivy like this simple oatmeal bath—and it does wonders on sunburns, rashes, and bug bites too. Oats relieve dryness, and baking soda exfoliates and helps balance your skin's pH level, while Atlas cedarwood essential oil neutralizes redness and delivers a calming aroma.

STEP 1 / Pulse the oats into a fine dust in a coffee grinder. Combine them with the baking soda in a bowl.

STEP 2 / Draw a warm (but not hot) bath and add ½ cup (45 g) of the oats and baking soda mixture. Stir to distribute.

STEP 3 / Combine the grape-seed oil and Atlas cedarwood essential oil in a small bowl, then either massage the blend into your skin or swirl it into your bathwater. (Don't add the oil until you've filled the tub, as some may evaporate with the hot water.)

STEP 4 / Relax in the bath for no more than 30 minutes. Get out and towel-dry, then generously apply a healing moisturizer like aloe vera or coconut oil.

Ever had a brother, husband, or male friend "borrow" your skincare products? Guys can have acne and oily skin too, and shaving can cause irritation or razor burn on top of it all. Cedarwood essential oil not only combats pimples, excess oil, and inflammation, it also gives skincare recipes an earthy, manly scent. These projects are easy to whip up, they smell amazing, and they make great gifts!

Brand-New-Day Aftershave

1 tablespoon witch hazel

1 teaspoon vegetable glycerin

½ teaspoon jojoba oil

5 drops Atlas cedarwood essential oil

3 drops sandalwood essential oil

1 drop cinnamon leaf essential oil

2-ounce (60-mL) glass bottle

2 tablespoons distilled water

Pour the witch hazel, vegetable glycerin, jojoba oil, and Atlas cedarwood, sandalwood, and cinnamon leaf essential oils into the bottle. Top it off with distilled water. Shake before every use, then rub 1 teaspoon between your palms and apply to your face and neck after shaving. Use within 3 months.

Conditioning Beard Oil

1 tablespoon whiskey

6 drops Atlas cedarwood essential oil

3 drops juniper berry essential oil

3 drops fir needle essential oil

2-ounce (60-mL) bottle

1 tablespoon argan oil

2 tablespoons grape-seed oil

Combine the whiskey and the Atlas cedarwood, juniper berry, and fir needle essential oils in your bottle. Add the argan and grape-seed oils, then shake. To use, agitate first to recombine the oils and whiskey, then pour about 1 teaspoon into the palm of your hand and stroke through a beard near you. Make sure to use within 6 months.

Aloe-Almond Facial Scrub

2 tablespoons almonds

2 tablespoons old-fashioned oats

2 tablespoons aloe vera gel

6 drops Atlas cedarwood essential oil

Pulse the almonds and oats in a coffee grinder until they're a fine powder. Transfer to a small bowl, then stir in the aloe vera gel and Atlas cedarwood essential oil. Massage into your face and let sit for 15 minutes, then remove with a warm washcloth. (Use this scrub before—not after—shaving, or on no-shave days.)

Cedarwood + Clay Man Mask

1 tablespoon red Moroccan clay

2 drops Atlas cedarwood essential oil

1 teaspoon apple cider vinegar

Combine the Moroccan clay, Atlas cedarwood essential oil, and apple cider vinegar in a small non-metal bowl, adding water as needed to create a paste. Apply to your face and let dry for 10 to 15 minutes. The superabsorbent red clay is great at extracting dirt from oily or acne-prone skin. Rinse with warm water.

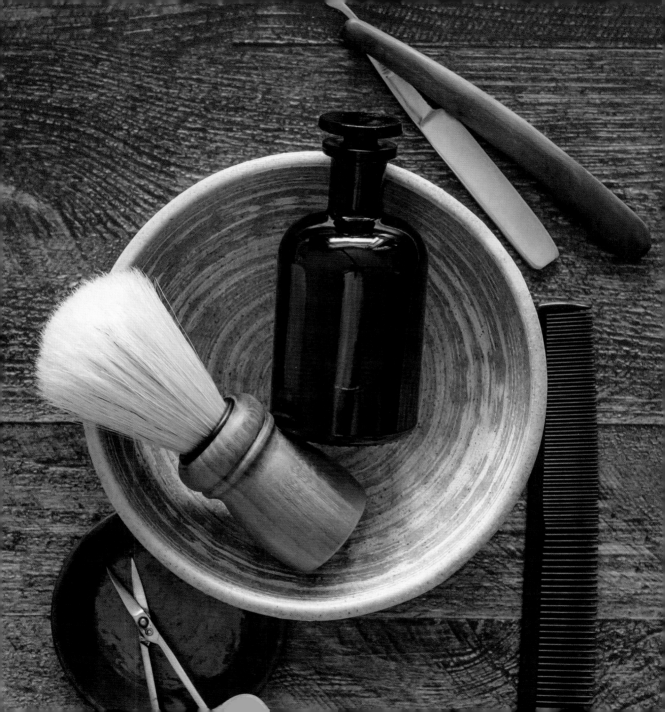

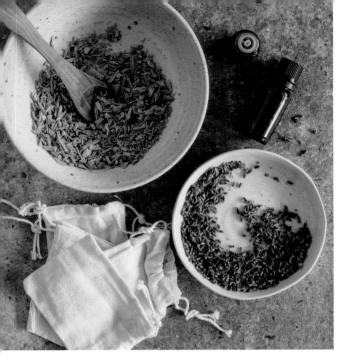
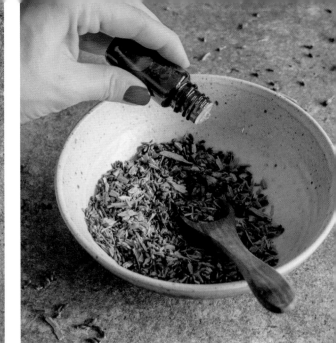
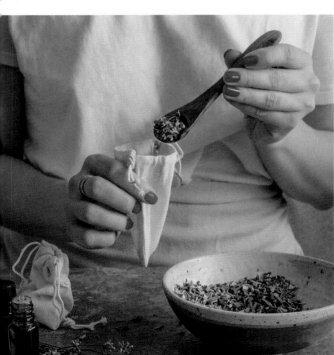
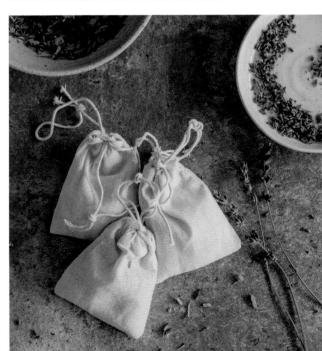

Protective Cedarwood Sachets

4 cups (360 g) cedarwood shavings

1 cup (40 g) dried lavender

20 drops Atlas cedarwood essential oil

18 drops lavender essential oil

5 to 7 3-by-5-inch (7.5-by-12.7-cm) muslin drawstring sachet bags

Replace nasty-smelling (and possibly carcinogenic) mothballs with naturally repellent DIY sachets. Atlas cedarwood guards your closet against moths and other insects; here it's paired with lavender for a floral note. Pour in the herbs, tie the sachet shut, and tuck it into closets and drawers for a fresh, foresty aroma.

STEP 1 / In a large mixing bowl, combine the cedarwood shavings and dried lavender. Sprinkle with the Atlas cedarwood and lavender essential oils, and mix together.

STEP 2 / Use a funnel to fill each sachet bag with ¾ cup (35 g) of the cedarwood-lavender mixture. (No bags? Place the shavings in the centers of fabric squares instead.)

STEP 3 / Cinch the bags shut, then squeeze them to crush the herbs and shavings and release their natural oils. (If using fabric squares, gather the corners and tie with string.)

STEP 4 / To use, place the sachets in a closet, drawer, or clothes hamper. If the scent starts to run out, simply open up the sachets and add more of the essential oils.

Citrus Rind + Salt Diffuser

1 whole grapefruit

1 cup (290 g) coarse sea salt

4 drops Atlas cedarwood essential oil

3 fresh sage leaves

These citrus-rind salt diffusers look cool while freshening up the air in your home, and they come together with just a few kitchen staples. The sea salt does double duty, absorbing bad odors from the environment while dispersing the Atlas cedarwood essential oil, fresh citrus, and herbaceous sage scents.

STEP 1 / Slice the grapefruit in half and carefully hollow out both sides using a paring knife and spoon.

STEP 2 / In a small bowl, mix the sea salt, Atlas cedarwood essential oil, and sage leaves together.

STEP 3 / Spoon the mixture into both halves of the grapefruit rind. Place each in a different room and enjoy the scent for a few days.

TIP / You can try a whole host of pleasant blends in simple citrus diffusers. For an orange-spice aroma, try mixing 5 drops cinnamon bark essential oil and 1 tablespoon whole cloves with ¾ cup (220 g) coarse sea salt, then place in 2 orange rinds. For a refreshing yet sweet scent, try blending 4 drops rosemary essential oil and 2 drops vanilla essential oil in ¾ cup (220 g) coarse sea salt, then distribute between 2 lemon rinds.

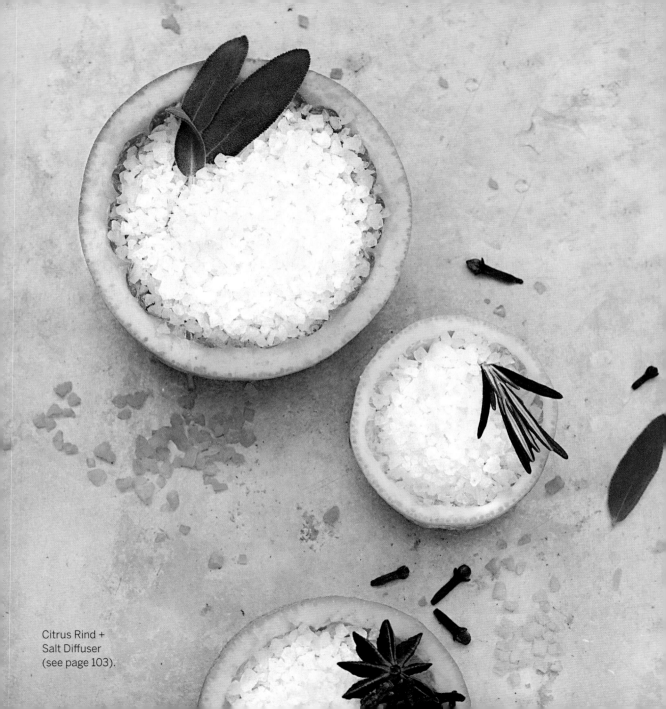

Citrus Rind +
Salt Diffuser
(see page 103).

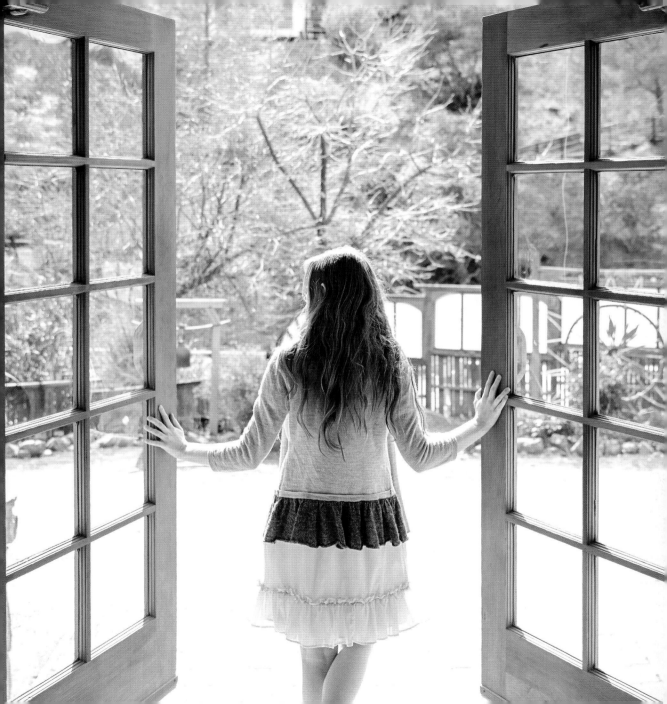

LEMONGRASS

This tropical grass is irrepressibly fragrant—it's lemony and earthy, refreshing and grounding. Chock-full of the antiseptic compound citral, lemongrass essential oil is a great choice for keeping infections at bay, fighting acne, and minimizing pores. When used in DIY cleaning recipes, its antimicrobial properties act as a natural sanitizer; when called on in soaps and deodorants, it vanquishes body odors. Related to palmarosa and citronella, lemongrass is a powerful insect repellent—and one you actually want to smell! In fact, inhaling this invigorating essential oil is known to improve concentration, boost energy, and ease headaches and jet lag.

Cymbopogon citratus | ORIGIN *Southeast Asia*

Pick-Me-Up Aromatherapy Inhaler

7 drops lemongrass essential oil
6 drops spearmint essential oil
5 drops melissa essential oil
3 drops sweet basil essential oil
Aromatherapy inhaler

Breathing in essential oils is one of the best ways to enjoy their benefits, but you can't exactly set up a diffuser at work or on a plane. Enter inhalers, pocket-size tubes that you can discreetly sniff when you need an aromatherapy treat. Try this breezy citrus and herb blend to boost brain function and revitalize your spirits.

STEP 1 / Drizzle the lemongrass, spearmint, melissa, and sweet basil essential oils into a small bowl. Remove the cap from the inhaler tube and pull out its cotton wick. Soak the wick in the oils for 1 to 2 minutes.

STEP 2 / Put the wick back inside the inhaler tube and replace the cap. Slide the cover over the tube, then label it for quick reference.

STEP 3 / Whenever you need to clear your mind, slide off the inhaler's cover and hold it close to your nose. Then try a little alternating nostril breathing: Press the right side of your nose closed with your thumb and breathe in through the left nostril. Exhale through the mouth and switch nostrils. Continue the breathing cycle until you feel energized and ready for whatever comes your way.

Bug-Banishing Spray

½ cup (120 mL) peppermint hydrosol (see page 16)
4-ounce (120-mL) spray bottle
16 drops lemongrass essential oil
14 drops lemon eucalyptus essential oil
12 drops Atlas cedarwood essential oil
10 drops geranium essential oil
10 drops lavender essential oil
10 drops tea tree essential oil

Fleas, lice, and ticks sure may not appreciate lemongrass, but kids and adults alike tend to enjoy its fresh, energizing scent. When teamed up with lemon eucalyptus, this homemade bug spray also deters mosquitoes and gnats—and creates a cooling sensation that's perfect for hot summer days.

STEP 1 / To make peppermint hydrosol, follow the instructions on page 16. (Or infuse ½ cup/15 g dried peppermint in 1 cup/240 mL witch hazel for 2 weeks. Strain well.)

STEP 2 / Pour ½ cup (120 mL) of the hydrosol or infused witch hazel into your bottle. Add the lemongrass, lemon eucalyptus, Atlas cedarwood, geranium, lavender, and tea tree essential oils. Replace the cap; shake.

STEP 3 / Agitate the bottle well before each application, then spray on any exposed skin before going outdoors. Reapply every 2 hours and use within 1 year.

TIP / Lemongrass essential oil is potent stuff. For topical applications, use a maximum of 4 drops for every 1 ounce carrier oil. Avoid overuse, and wash it off with soap and water if an adverse reaction occurs.

Rainbow Dream Bath Bombs

½ cup (60 g) citric acid

1 cup (220 g) baking soda

½ cup (60 g) cornstarch

½ cup (120 g) Epsom salt

12 drops lemongrass
essential oil

83 drops lavender essential oil

12 drops Roman chamomile
essential oil

24 drops clary sage essential oil

1 teaspoon sweet almond oil

3 tablespoons coconut oil

Natural food coloring in 3 colors
of your choosing

Mold

Mica (optional)

No matter how chaotic life gets, you can always count on a warm bath! Beyond calming sore muscles and cramps, a bath is a great way to soak away a stressful day and turn a foul mood around. These bath bombs deliver the moisturizing goods (in the form of two lightweight oils) and a revitalizing, balancing blend of essential oils. Lemongrass cleanses emotional turmoil to promote confidence, while lavender, clary sage, and Roman chamomile ease anxiety and irritability.

STEP 1 / In a large bowl, combine the dry ingredients: the citric acid, baking soda, cornstarch, and Epsom salt. Stir to combine, breaking up any clumps.

STEP 2 / Combine the lemongrass, lavender, Roman chamomile, and clary sage essential oils with the sweet almond oil in a small measuring cup with a spout.

STEP 3 / Pour the essential oil mixture into the bowl of dry ingredients, then mix thoroughly. Divide the mixture into three smaller bowls.

STEP 4 / In the microwave, melt 1 tablespoon coconut oil in a spouted heat-safe glass measuring cup for 10 seconds. Continue with 5-second blasts until it's fully melted, stirring in between each.

STEP 5 / Add 2 drops of your first natural food coloring to the melted coconut oil. Pour the oil into one of the three bowls and use your hands to mix the contents together. Adjust the color, if desired.

STEP 6 / Repeat steps 4 and 5 with a different color. Repeat a third time so each bowl of dry ingredients has been thoroughly mixed with a different color of the oil mixture.

STEP 7 / Pack the mixtures into whatever mold you like, layering the colors on top of each other and along the sides of the mold. (If using a ball mold, as shown here, pack each side until overflowing, and squeeze both halves together to close.) This recipe will yield four bath bombs.

STEP 8 / Freeze for 20 minutes before use. To remove a bath bomb from the mold, warm the sides of the mold with your hands (this will help melt the coconut oil) and squeeze either side until the bomb pops out. Sprinkle with mica for a little shimmer, if desired.

STEP 9 / To use, fill your tub with warm water and drop in a bath bomb. It will fizz, releasing its scent and all its skin-softening agents. Soak for 20 to 30 minutes. Store in an airtight container and use within 6 months.

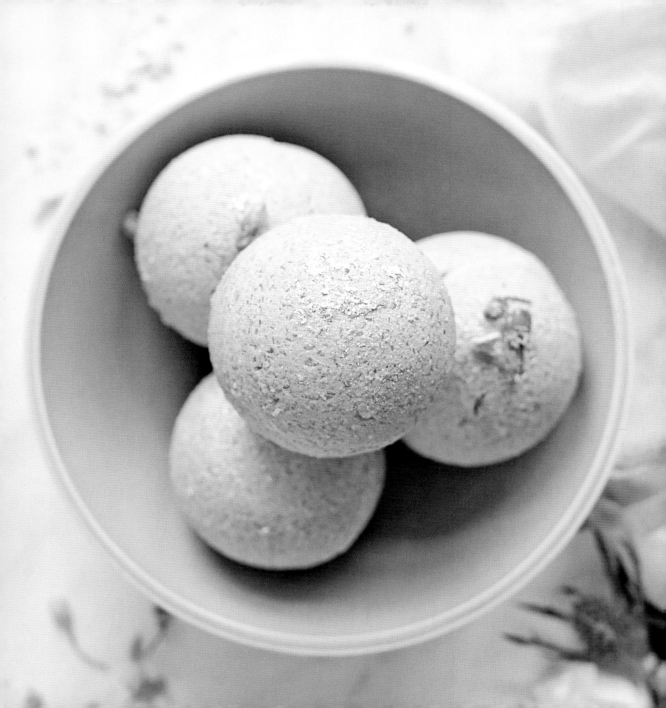

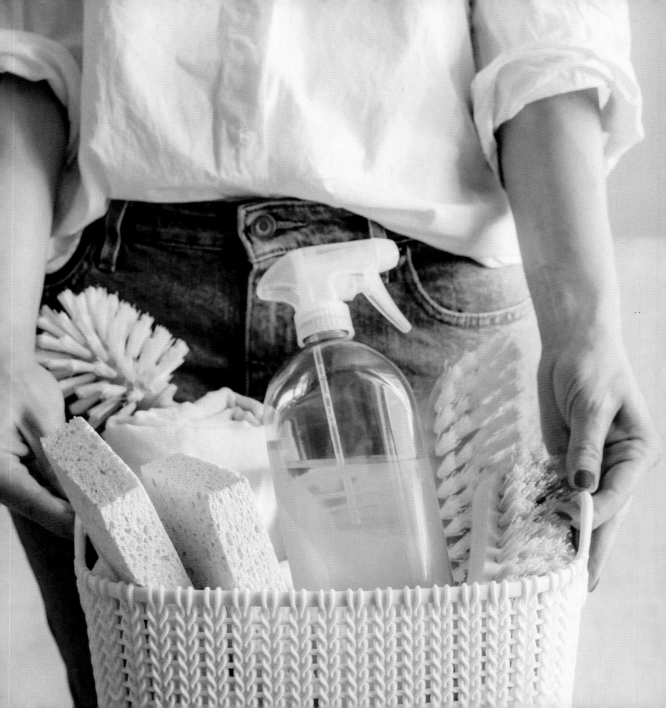

Lemon-Thyme All-Purpose Spray

2 lemons

Several sprigs of fresh thyme

16-ounce (475-mL) jar

2 cups (475 mL) distilled
white vinegar

20-ounce (590-mL) spray bottle

2 cups (475 mL) distilled water

20 drops lemongrass
essential oil

10 drops lemon essential oil

10 drops thyme essential oil

Vinegar is nature's all-purpose cleaner, but—as you're probably aware—it totally stinks. If you infuse it, however, you can add natural cleansing and disinfecting benefits while creating a much more pleasant aromatherapy experience. Try lemon, thyme, and lemongrass essential oils, and you've got a go-to cleaning spray that's all natural and makes your house smell better—not worse!

STEP 1 / Using a knife, cut the peel from the lemons and scrape off as much pith as you can. Place the lemon peels and thyme sprigs inside your jar.

STEP 2 / Fill the jar with the distilled white vinegar and replace the lid. Give the jar a good shake to coat the infusion ingredients.

STEP 3 / Here's where patience is a virtue. Find a sunny spot and let the oils from the lemons and thyme infuse the vinegar for 10 to 14 days.

STEP 4 / After the infusion period has ended, filter out the solids from the vinegar using a fine-mesh strainer and discard them.

STEP 5 / Pour ½ cup (120 mL) of the infused vinegar into a spray bottle. (Return the extra vinegar to your infusion jar until needed.)

STEP 6 / Add the distilled water and the lemongrass, lemon, and thyme essential oils to the spray bottle. (If your bottle is bigger than 20 ounces/590 mL, increase the amounts of the ingredients while keeping the same 4:1 ratio of water to infused vinegar.) Swirl to blend the ingredients together.

STEP 7 / To use, first agitate to remix the oils, then spray onto countertops, sinks, and toilets. Wipe down with a wet rag. (Note: Don't use this cleaner on marble, as vinegar can erode the stone.) Store in a cool, dark spot, and use within 3 months.

TIP / If lemons aren't your thing, go wild and create your own blend with cinnamon sticks, whole cloves, orange peels, eucalyptus leaves, or whatever herbs you have on hand.

Focus + Memory

Essential oils can come in handy when you're prepping for an important presentation or studying for an exam—they can even give you a memory assist when the big day comes. Use these blends to stay focused the next time you need to fight fatigue, control stress levels, and ace whatever's on your plate.

GAME-DAY DE-STRESS DIFFUSER

Let these refreshingly herbaceous essential oils inspire you to excel at work or school. Just add them to an electric diffuser when you need a little motivation—consider it a pep talk for your nose! Scale the volume of oils as needed for your diffuser model.

TAKE-A-BREAK BATH SALTS

When you need a breather, consider soaking in a relaxing bath to reduce exhaustion and improve mental clarity. Mix these essential oils with 1 tablespoon carrier oil and dissolve into ½ cup (145 g) sea salts. Add to a warm bath and soak for 30 minutes.

INVIGORATING BODY WASH

This pick-me-up body wash is designed to stimulate, focus, and refresh your mind. Mix ½ cup (120 mL) unscented liquid castile soap with ¼ cup (60 mL) each grape-seed oil and honey in a bowl. Add the essential oils below and pour into a pump bottle.

Cinnamon Leaf
3 drops

Thyme
1 drop

Rosemary
4 drops

Pine
2 drops

Peppermint
15 drops

Lime
9 drops

Grapefruit
3 drops

Peppermint
3 drops

Spruce
2 drops

Sandalwood
2 drops

Black Pepper
6 drops

TENSION-RELIEF ROLLERBALL

Intense concentration can trigger tension. Add these essential oils to a 10-mL roll-on applicator, then fill the rest of the tube with a carrier oil of your choosing. Apply to your forehead and behind the ears when stress hits, then give yourself a temple massage.

ON-TASK REFOCUSING MIST

When your mind starts to wander, get it back on track by spritzing this revitalizing blend over your desk—it'll improve concentration and step up your mood. To make, add these essential oils to a spray bottle with 4 ounces (120 mL) water.

CONCENTRATION-BOOST SMELLING SALTS BOWL

Combine these essential oils with 2 tablespoons salt in a small decorative bowl and place it at your work station. Inhale the scent whenever you feel your attention start to wane for an instant perk-up.

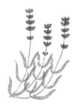
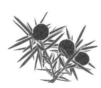

Lavender
6 drops

Juniper Berry
2 drops

Bergamot
75 drops

Clary Sage
50 drops

Pine
10 drops

Hyssop
5 drops

Rosemary
4 drops

Frankincense
25 drops

Eucalyptus
5 drops

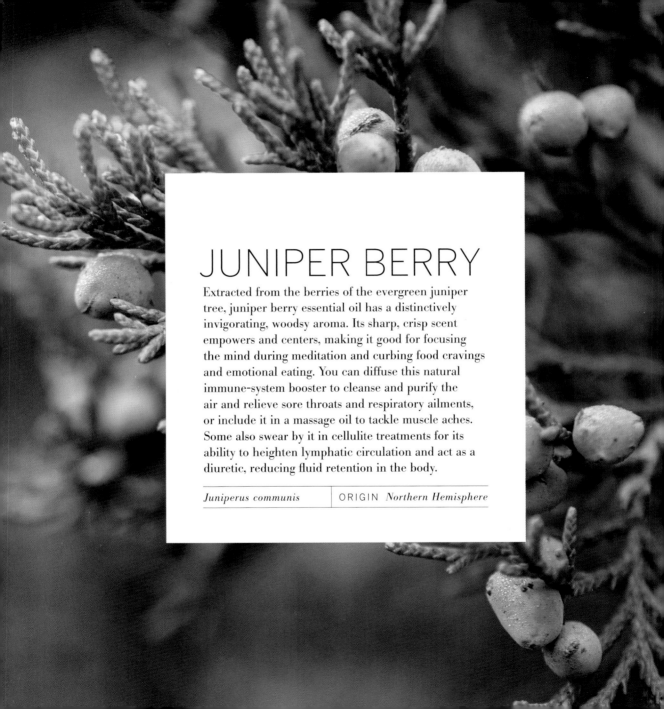

JUNIPER BERRY

Extracted from the berries of the evergreen juniper tree, juniper berry essential oil has a distinctively invigorating, woodsy aroma. Its sharp, crisp scent empowers and centers, making it good for focusing the mind during meditation and curbing food cravings and emotional eating. You can diffuse this natural immune-system booster to cleanse and purify the air and relieve sore throats and respiratory ailments, or include it in a massage oil to tackle muscle aches. Some also swear by it in cellulite treatments for its ability to heighten lymphatic circulation and act as a diuretic, reducing fluid retention in the body.

Juniperus communis | ORIGIN *Northern Hemisphere*

All-Purpose Aromatherapy Oil

2 tablespoons carrier oil, such
as sweet almond, apricot kernel,
sesame, or grape-seed

4 drops juniper berry
essential oil

2 drops grapefruit essential oil

1 drop cypress essential oil

1 drop lemon essential oil

1 drop sweet orange essential oil

1-ounce (30-mL) dark glass
bottle

This extra-easy "everything oil" is a godsend: It's perfect as an after-shower moisturizer, in a relaxing evening bath, or as part of your dry-brushing routine. One of its best uses, however, is as a stress-busting massage oil. Combine all the benefits of massage—improved circulation, relieved tension, and released toxins—with the insomnia-easing, anxiety-reducing aromatherapy benefits of juniper berry essential oil, and your mind and body will be all the better for it.

STEP 1 / Pour your favorite carrier oil into a spouted measuring cup.

STEP 2 / Slowly drizzle in the juniper berry, grapefruit, cypress, lemon, and sweet orange essential oils.

STEP 3 / Pour the oil mixture carefully into your dark bottle and shake well to combine. Label the bottle—trust me, you won't remember what's in there!

STEP 4 / To use, agitate and pour 1 teaspoon into your hands. Massage into your skin with upward-circular movements. And no, there's no masseuse required for at-home massages—try rubbing your own temples, hands, legs, feet, or face.

TIP / To stimulate the lymphatic system and improve circulation, apply 1 to 2 drops to a dry brush and, starting at your feet, sweep up toward your heart.

MORE MASSAGE OIL COMBOS

Massage has many benefits, including improving circulation, easing tension, and stimulating the body to discharge toxins. When you combine it with aromatherapy, a happy synergy happens. Try your own blends by adding 6 to 12 drops essential oil for every 1 ounce (30 mL) carrier oil, such as sweet almond, apricot kernel, or grape-seed. Here are some starter ideas.

REFRESHING 4 drops each lemon, sweet basil, and peppermint.

RELAXING HAND 3 drops neroli, 2 drops frankincense, 2 drops bergamot, 2 drops sweet orange, and 1 drop sandalwood.

BRAIN-POWER 6 drops peppermint and 4 drops rosemary.

DE-STRESS 5 drops clary sage, 4 drops bergamot, and 2 drops lavender.

FACE-CALMING 3 drops rose absolute, 3 drops frankincense, 2 drops geranium, and 2 drops carrot-seed.

HANGOVER CURE 4 drops juniper berry, 3 drops geranium, 3 drops cardamom, and 2 drops lavender.

Head-to-Toe Clay Body Mask

½ cup (70 g) bentonite clay

2 tablespoons sea salt
(or Epsom salt)

¼ cup (60 mL) castor oil

¼ cup (60 mL) aloe vera gel

24 drops juniper berry
essential oil

10 drops peppermint
essential oil

It wouldn't be a spa day without a body wrap, but you can make this splurge on the cheap at home. Clay is a great skin detoxer, while juniper berry essential oil reduces water retention and can help improve the appearance of cellulite. Add bloat-beating castor oil for an experience that pampers and perks you right up.

STEP 1 / Mix the bentonite clay and salt in a bowl. (Don't use metal tools, as they can deactivate the clay.)

STEP 2 / Warm the castor oil to boost its liver-detoxing, stretchmark-smoothing abilities, then add it to the aloe vera gel. (If you're pregnant or menstruating, swap the castor oil with a hydrating oil, like coconut, almond, or grape-seed.)

STEP 3 / Drizzle in the juniper berry and peppermint essential oils, then

stir with a wooden spoon. If the mixture is too thick, add water until it's smooth and easily spreadable.

STEP 4 / Standing on a sheet or in the tub, apply a thin layer of the mixture to your skin. Start with your feet and work your way up, ending with your arms and hands.

STEP 5 / Wrap up in a warm towel or bedsheet and relax for 1 hour. Rinse off the mixture with warm water, and follow up with moisturizer.

Cafe Mocha Scrub Bars

½ cup (50 g) coconut oil

2 tablespoons shea butter

½ cup (100 g) fresh, unused coffee grounds

2 tablespoons cocoa powder

24 drops juniper berry
essential oil

It seems there's always a new study claiming coffee and chocolate are good for us—turns out it's true in the beauty world! Cocoa powder's antioxidants help fix skin damage caused by the sun, while coffee exfoliates to reveal baby-soft skin.

STEP 1 / Bring 2 inches (5 cm) of water to a boil in a small saucepan. Mix the coconut oil and shea butter in a heat-safe glass bowl. Place it over the saucepan and turn the heat to low, stirring until the mixture melts.

STEP 2 / Remove from the heat. Add the coffee grounds, cocoa powder, and juniper berry essential oil.

STEP 3 / Spoon into an ice cube tray and freeze.

STEP 4 / Remove 1 cube and let it soften for 5 minutes. Rub over your skin in circular motions in the shower, then rinse. Let the warm water run for 3 minutes to rinse the scrub down the drain. Store the rest in a plastic bag in the freezer; use within 6 months.

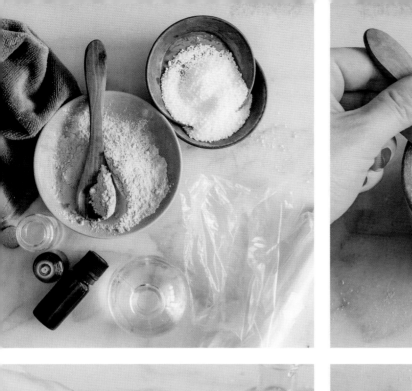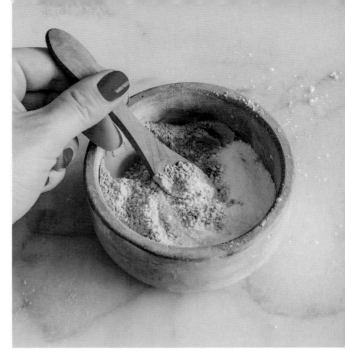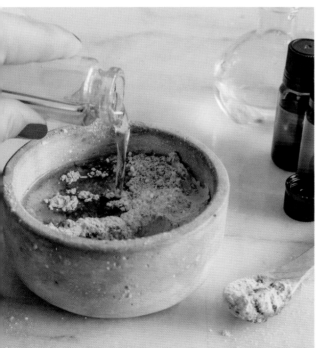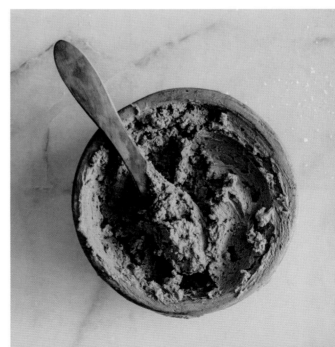

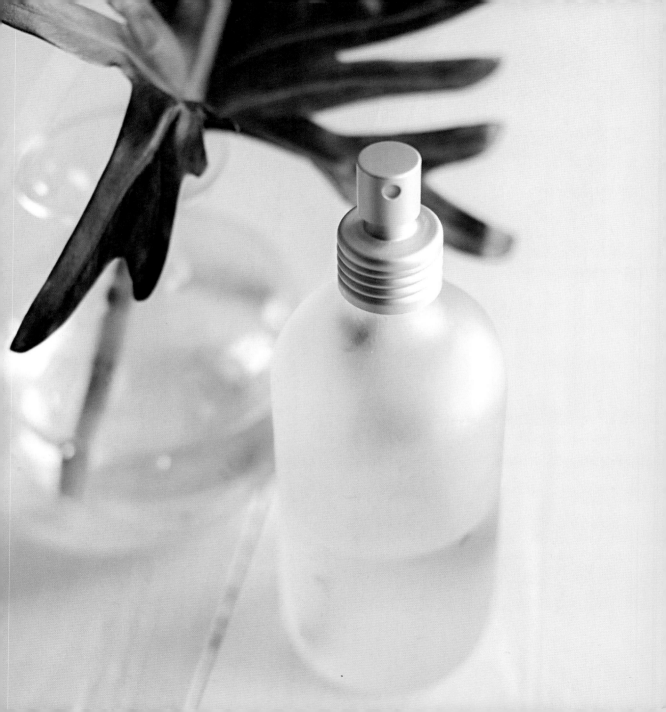

Green Earth Room Spray

2 tablespoons vodka or
witch hazel

2-ounce (60-mL) glass
spray bottle

30 drops juniper berry
essential oil

20 drops rosemary essential oil

13 drops frankincense
essential oil

12 drops jasmine essential oil

2 tablespoons distilled water

Capture all the invigorating vibes of spring with this upbeat, cleansing, and purifying room spray—one spritz and you'll be seeing visions of freshly mowed grass, new buds on trees, longer days, and plenty of sunshine ahead. The spring scents (including essential oils that both boost energy and beat anxiety) will energize you and help jump-start spring-cleaning tasks. They'll also hydrate the air, which is often dry after running the heat during the winter.

STEP 1 / Pour the alcohol or witch hazel into the spray bottle. Add the juniper berry, rosemary, frankincense, and jasmine essential oils.

STEP 2 / Replace the bottle cap and swirl to combine the alcohol and oils. Allow the essential oils to dissolve in the alcohol for 20 minutes, then pour in the distilled water and replace the cap. Shake again.

STEP 3 / Give the bottle a quick shake before each use and then mist rooms throughout your home. Use within 3 months.

TIP / Don't like jasmine's sweetness? Try sunny grapefruit or bergamot, or a woodsy scent like pine or cypress.

Carpet Cure-All Treatment

2 cups (180 g) baking soda

½ cup (65 g) cornstarch

1 tablespoon unscented castile
soap flakes

20 drops juniper berry
essential oil

10 drops lemon essential oil

20-ounce (590-mL) container

With foot traffic and pets, it's easy for carpets to get dingy and a bit smelly. Skip the steam cleaner and make your own deodorizing carpet cleaner. Baking soda and cornstarch absorb odors and lift grease and grime, while mighty soap flakes tackle tough stains. Juniper and lemon essential oils leave a fresh, clean scent.

STEP 1 / Combine the baking soda, cornstarch, unscented castile soap flakes, and juniper berry and lemon essential oils in a mixing bowl. Use a fork to break up any clumps.

STEP 2 / Transfer the baking soda mixture to your container.

STEP 3 / Before use on carpets or rugs, test it on an inconspicuous spot for discoloration. Shake a thin layer onto your carpet; scrub any stains with a soft cloth. Let the mixture sit for 20 minutes, then vacuum it all up.

STEP 4 / Store in a cool, dry spot; use within 6 months.

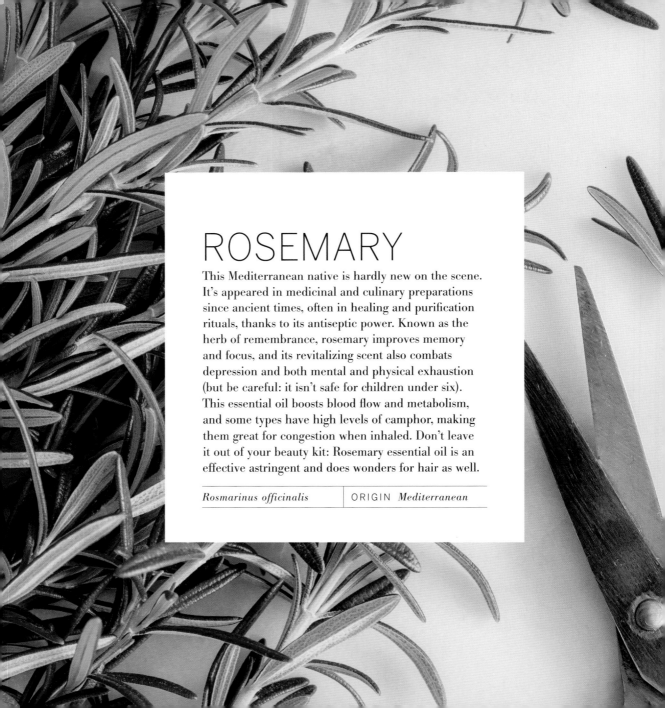

ROSEMARY

This Mediterranean native is hardly new on the scene. It's appeared in medicinal and culinary preparations since ancient times, often in healing and purification rituals, thanks to its antiseptic power. Known as the herb of remembrance, rosemary improves memory and focus, and its revitalizing scent also combats depression and both mental and physical exhaustion (but be careful: it isn't safe for children under six). This essential oil boosts blood flow and metabolism, and some types have high levels of camphor, making them great for congestion when inhaled. Don't leave it out of your beauty kit: Rosemary essential oil is an effective astringent and does wonders for hair as well.

Rosmarinus officinalis | ORIGIN *Mediterranean*

Heavy-Duty Laundry Detergent

2 laundry soap bars

4 soap bars

2 cups (560 g) super washing soda

2 cups (820 g) borax

25 drops rosemary essential oil

15 drops tea tree essential oil

3-quart (3-L) glass jar

If your clothes keep coming out less than clean, DIY this superpowered laundry detergent, which harnesses the antibacterial, antifungal, antiseptic, and antiviral properties of rosemary essential oil (with a little help from tea tree, of course).

STEP 1 / Grate all the soaps with a food processor's grating disk. Switch to the blade and pulse into a powder.

STEP 2 / Add the super washing soda, borax, and rosemary and tea tree essential oils to the food processor; pulse until blended. Pour into your airtight glass jar.

STEP 3 / Use 1 tablespoon detergent for a regular load of laundry, 2 for a large one. If the detergent doesn't fully dissolve, try dissolving it in 1 cup (240 mL) of warm water before adding it to the wash. Adding 1 cup (240 mL) of vinegar will also act as a natural softener and rinse away soap residue. Use within 1 year.

TIP / For a big batch of liquid detergent, mix all the powder with 2 gallons (7.5 L) plus 1 quart (1 L) of hot water in a 5-gallon (20-L) bucket. Use 1 cup (240 mL) liquid detergent per load. (Note that the liquid will be thicker than store-bought liquid detergent.)

Cozy Rosemary-Spice Fire Starters

½ cup (60 g) dried orange, grapefruit, and apple peels

½ tablespoon whole cloves

1 cinnamon stick

4 sprigs fresh rosemary

2 tablespoons dried lavender

10 drops rosemary essential oil

8 drops sweet orange essential oil

2 drops cinnamon leaf or bark essential oil

2 to 4 cone-shape coffee filters

12 inches (30 cm) embroidery thread and needle

Even if it doesn't reach subzero temperatures where you live, there's nothing like a heavenly scented fire to make you feel all warm and cozy. These fire starters take just minutes to make, and they're a great way to use up spices, coffee filters, and all that extra embroidery thread taking up space in your craft drawer too.

STEP 1 / Put the dried orange, grapefruit, and apple peels in a bowl, then add the cloves, cinnamon stick, rosemary, and dried lavender. (You can break the cinnamon stick into smaller pieces.)

STEP 2 / Stir in the rosemary, sweet orange, and cinnamon leaf or bark essential oils.

STEP 3 / Scoop up about ¼ cup (10 g) of the mixture and pour it into each coffee filter.

STEP 4 / Thread the needle and sew the top of each coffee filter closed. To use, simply toss one in the fire and enjoy the scrumptious warmth.

Hair-product ads are always touting the latest magical—though supposedly scientific—volume-boosting, shine-enhancing ingredients. Want to know the real go-to for great hair? Rosemary. Because it boosts blood flow, this herb promotes hair growth, slows graying, and reduces buildup, leaving you with thick, bouncy, glossy locks. Try these DIY hair remedies for all the good stuff without the harsh chemicals, hormone disrupters, and heavy metals found in store-bought products.

Guinness Volumizing Rinse

1 can Guinness (or other strong ale or stout)	5 drops rosemary essential oil

Open the beer and add the rosemary essential oil, then let the beer sit open overnight or until flat. After shampooing, rinse your hair with the beer. (I find it more pleasant to bend over and pour the cold brew forward over my hair instead of down my back.) Let the rinse sit for 5 minutes, massaging it into the roots of your hair. Rinse and style as usual.

Nourishing Rosemary-Yogurt Hair Mask

1 cup (245 g) organic full-fat plain yogurt	10 drops rosemary essential oil
1 tablespoon honey	1 teaspoon jojoba oil

Mix the yogurt, honey, rosemary essential oil, and jojoba oil in a small bowl. Coat your hair in the mixture, beginning with the ends and working up to your scalp. Pop on a shower cap and let the mixture soak in for 30 minutes, then hop in the shower to rinse it out. Shampoo and condition as usual.

Strengthening Nettle Tea Treatment

1 cup (240 mL) distilled water	1 nettle tea bag
¾ cup (20 g) fresh rosemary	5 drops rosemary essential oil

Bring the distilled water to a boil and add the fresh rosemary and nettle tea bag. Remove from the heat; let steep for 1 hour. Strain and allow to cool, then drizzle in the rosemary essential oil. Pour the mixture over your hair, combing through to saturate your strands. Let sit for 10 minutes, then rinse and shampoo as normal. (Tip: You can also pour the mixture into a spray bottle, spritz on wet hair, and leave on overnight.) Refrigerate any leftovers; use within 2 weeks.)

Simple DIY Detangling Spray

2 tablespoons all-natural conditioner	1 cup (240 mL) warm distilled water
8-ounce (240-mL) spray bottle	6 drops rosemary essential oil

Add the all-natural conditioner of your choice to your spray bottle, then fill the bottle with the warm distilled water and replace the cap. Shake to mix well and dissolve the conditioner, then add the rosemary essential oil and shake again. To use, spritz the mixture onto your hair and comb out the tangles, starting with the ends. Be sure to use within 3 months.

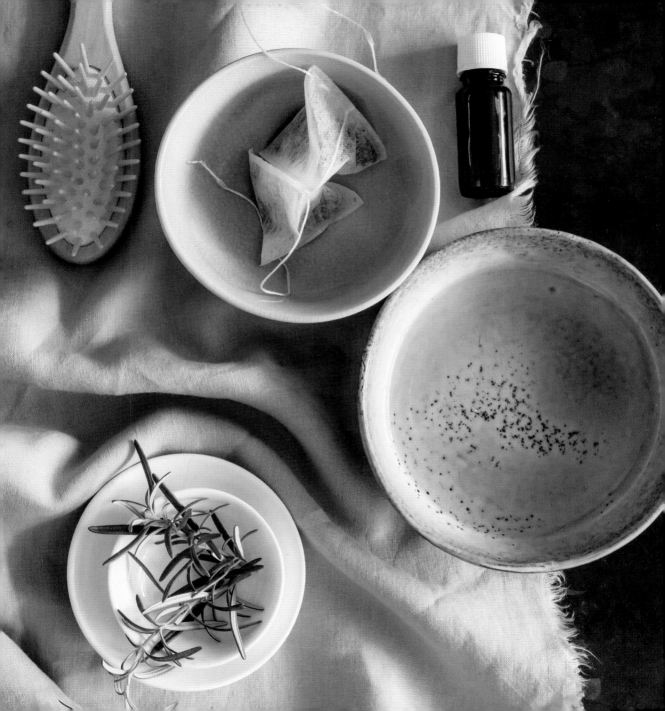

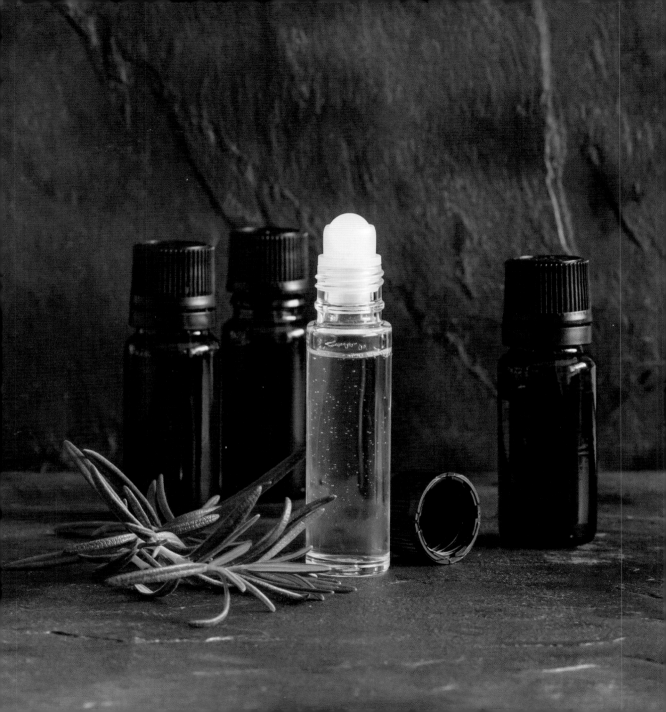

Headache Relief Roll-On

10-mL roll-on applicator,
preferably in dark glass

6 drops rosemary essential oil

4 drops lemon essential oil

2 drops peppermint essential oil

⅓ ounce (10 mL) carrier oil,
such as fractionated coconut,
olive, jojoba, or sweet almond

Essential oils have so many practical uses, but they can be tricky to apply. That's why these handy little rollerball bottles are a lifesaver: They're portable and dead simple to use. This particular roll-on contains rosemary, lemon, and peppermint—a blend that dulls pain, clears your mind, and helps you focus.

STEP 1 / Remove the rollerball from the top of the bottle and drizzle the rosemary, lemon, and peppermint essential oils into the bottle.

STEP 2 / Fill the bottle with the carrier oil of your choosing and pop the rollerball back in the applicator.

STEP 3 / Before each use, first roll the bottle between your hands to ensure the essential oils are properly mixed. Then apply to pressure points all over the body, such as the temples, behind the ears, bottoms of the feet, and insides of the wrists.

STEP 4 / Store your roll-on applicator in a cool, dark place—like your desk drawer for deadline-induced migraines or your glove compartment for traffic annoyances.

Take-the-Sting-Out Black Salve

½ cup (120 mL) calendula-
infused oil (see page 16)

2 teaspoons beeswax pellets

16 drops rosemary essential oil

16 drops lavender essential oil

16 drops tea tree essential oil

3 teaspoons activated charcoal
(approximately 15 capsules)

3 teaspoons bentonite clay

½ teaspoon vitamin E oil

4-ounce (120-mL) glass jar

Activated charcoal is great for stings, itches, and splinters—and for making a real mess. The good news is that this salve gives you all the relief without the need for cleanup. Its other ingredients are must-haves in any natural-remedy kit: The clay detoxes the skin while the antibacterial essential oils help prevent infection.

STEP 1 / Follow the steps on page 16 to make calendula-infused oil.

STEP 2 / Combine the calendula oil and beeswax pellets in a heat-safe glass bowl. Bring 2 inches (5 cm) of water to a bowl in a saucepan, then place the bowl on top and heat on low.

STEP 3 / When the beeswax has melted, remove the mixture from the heat. Add the rosemary, lavender, and tea tree essential oils. Let the oil continue to cool for 2 to 3 minutes.

STEP 4 / Stir in the activated charcoal, bentonite clay, and vitamin E oil with a wooden or plastic spoon. Transfer to your jar and let set.

STEP 5 / Apply to bug bites, stings, or splinters and cover with a bandage, reapplying every 12 hours as needed. Store in a cool spot; use within 1 year.

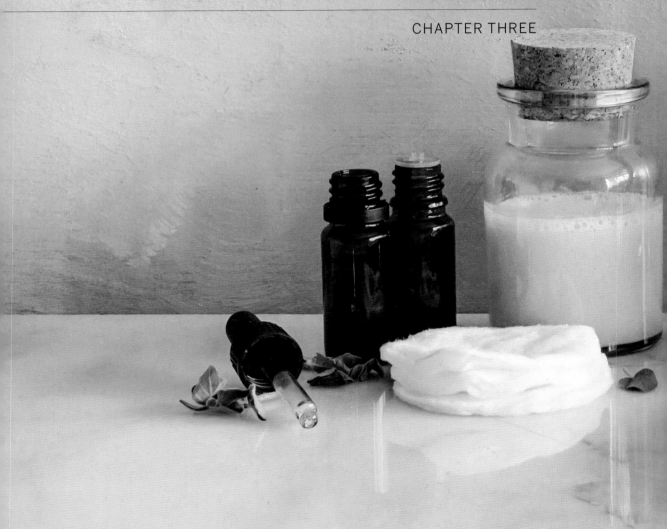

Restore

CHAPTER THREE

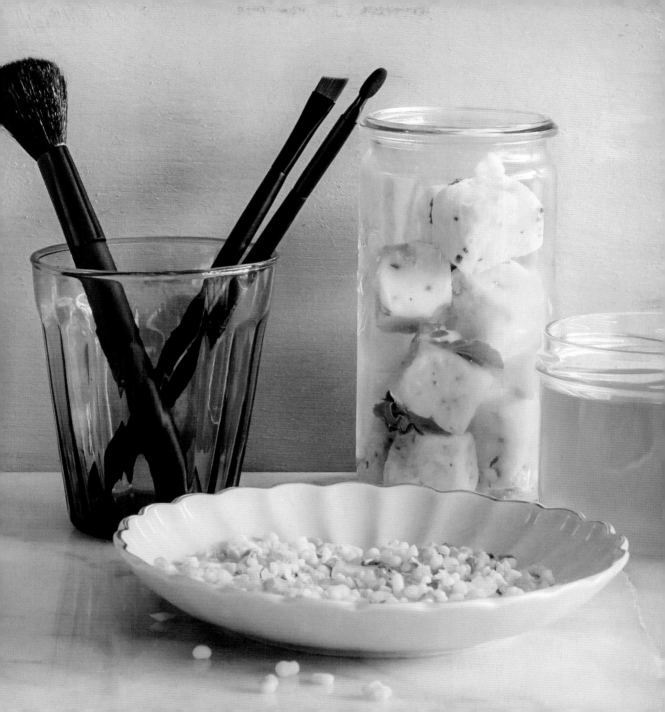

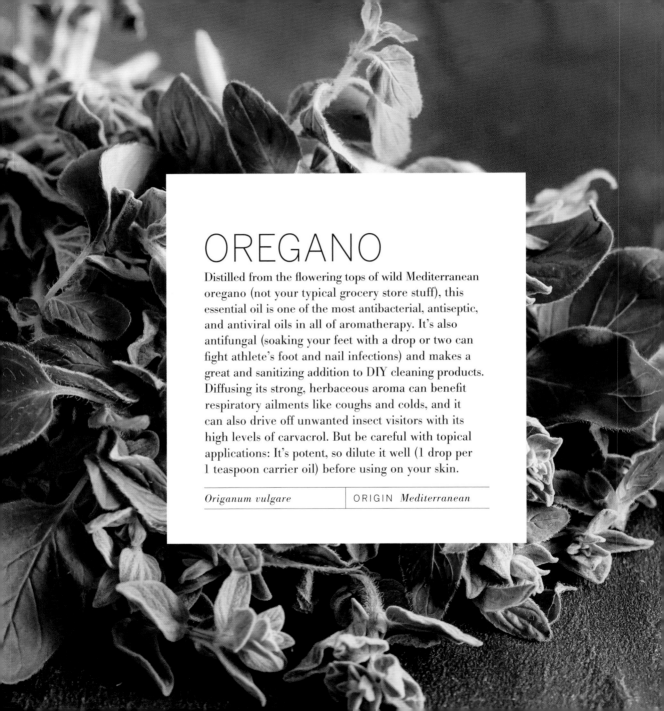

OREGANO

Distilled from the flowering tops of wild Mediterranean oregano (not your typical grocery store stuff), this essential oil is one of the most antibacterial, antiseptic, and antiviral oils in all of aromatherapy. It's also antifungal (soaking your feet with a drop or two can fight athlete's foot and nail infections) and makes a great and sanitizing addition to DIY cleaning products. Diffusing its strong, herbaceous aroma can benefit respiratory ailments like coughs and colds, and it can also drive off unwanted insect visitors with its high levels of carvacrol. But be careful with topical applications: It's potent, so dilute it well (1 drop per 1 teaspoon carrier oil) before using on your skin.

Origanum vulgare | ORIGIN *Mediterranean*

Make-It-Sparkle Sink Scrub

1 cup (220 g) baking soda

1 heaping tablespoon
dried oregano

1 heaping tablespoon
dried thyme

1 heaping tablespoon
dried rosemary

5 drops thyme essential oil

3 drops oregano essential oil

2 tablespoons borax
(optional)

10-ounce (295-mL)
airtight container

Scrubbing the sink is no fun, but it's better with products you like. Baking soda is Mother Nature's scouring powder and, combined with herbs and spices, it might even make you look forward to your date with porcelain. Keep a large batch in an airtight container in the kitchen or bathroom, and shake it over surfaces whenever you want—you'll be left with a sparkling sink and an amazing smell.

STEP 1 / Combine the baking soda, oregano, thyme, and rosemary in a food processor. Pulse until the herbs are finely ground.

STEP 2 / Add the thyme and oregano essential oils; pulse again. For extra stain-fighting power, add 2 tablespoons borax.

STEP 3 / Transfer the mixture to your container and sprinkle onto bathroom and kitchen surfaces, then scrub with a damp cloth or sponge. Rinse well with water, and you're good to go. Use within 1 year.

Mold + Mildew Shower Spray

16-ounce (475-mL) spray bottle

2 cups (475 mL) distilled
white vinegar

1 teaspoon tea tree essential oil

20 drops oregano essential oil

10 drops sweet orange
essential oil

If your bathroom lacks a window, you know that the mildew struggle is real. This DIY spray smells better than bleach, and it harnesses the disinfecting power of vinegar and essential oils to make a cheap, safe cleaner that actually gets rid of soap scum and mildew—and prevents mold from occurring in the first place.

STEP 1 / Fill the spray bottle with the distilled white vinegar and the tea tree, oregano, and sweet orange essential oils.

STEP 2 / Saturate any moldy areas with the mixture and let it dry. Porous surfaces will absorb the spray, allowing it to kill mold beneath the surface—something bleach can't do!

STEP 3 / Put on a pair of gloves and scrub off all the mold stains.

STEP 4 / Wet a rag with the solution and wipe the surface to remove any residual mold and spores, then spray the area again without rinsing to help prevent a mold comeback.

STEP 5 / To keep your bathroom mold and mildew free, spray your shower daily and let it dry. Since vinegar and oil don't mix well, shake the bottle well before each use. Store in a cool, dark spot; use within 1 year.

Breath-of-Fresh-Air Mouthwash

1 drop oregano essential oil
prediluted in olive oil

2 drops peppermint essential oil

8-ounce (240-mL) glass bottle

1 cup (240 mL) distilled water

2 teaspoons baking soda

1 teaspoon trace mineral drops

5 drops liquid stevia (optional)

Don't believe the ads: That burning sensation caused by those neon green, chemical-laden, store-bought mouthwashes is in no way good for you. Get that squeaky-clean feeling from this homemade mouthwash instead! The peppermint and oregano essential oils work hard to combat bacteria, plaque, and bad breath, while baking soda helps remove stains and whiten teeth.

STEP 1 / Drizzle the oregano and peppermint essential oils into your glass bottle. Pour in the distilled water and baking soda.

STEP 2 / Add the trace mineral drops, which will help replenish mineral stores in your teeth and gums.

STEP 3 / Use the mouthwash in the morning and at night after brushing your teeth. (If you need a little sweetness, add a drop or two of liquid stevia.) Do not swallow.

TIP / While the essential oils inhibit bacteria growth, make a fresh batch every week to avoid contamination.

All-Natural Hand Sanitizer

1 teaspoon vegetable glycerin

2 ounces (60 mL) witch hazel

2 tablespoons aloe vera gel

13 drops lemon essential oil

13 drops sweet orange
essential oil

9 drops oregano essential oil
prediluted in olive oil

4-ounce (120-mL) spray bottle

Hand sanitizer may seem like a necessary evil, but you can skip those alcohol-based gels, which smell horrible, contain nasty ingredients, dry out your hands, and—wait for it—are no more effective than washing with soap and water. Try this gentle homemade version, which gets its mighty cleansing power and refreshing scent from antibacterial lemon, oregano, and tea tree essential oils.

STEP 1 / Combine the vegetable glycerin, witch hazel, and aloe vera gel in a small measuring cup.

STEP 2 / Add the lemon, sweet orange, and oregano essential oils.

STEP 3 / Pour the mixture into your spray bottle. Add the cap and give it a good shake.

STEP 4 / To apply, just give your hands 2 to 3 sprays and rub together. The ingredients tend to separate between uses, so give the bottle a gentle shake before each application. Keep in your car or purse for easy on-the-go access. Be sure to use within 6 months.

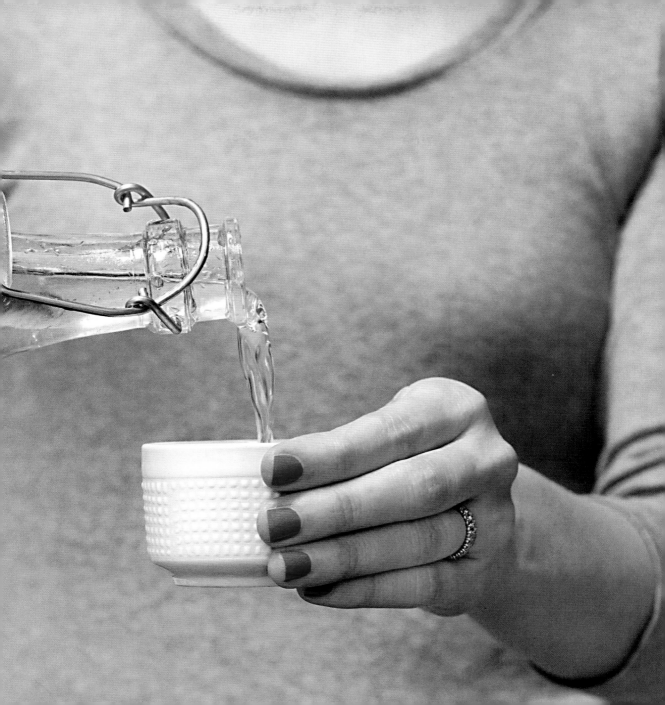

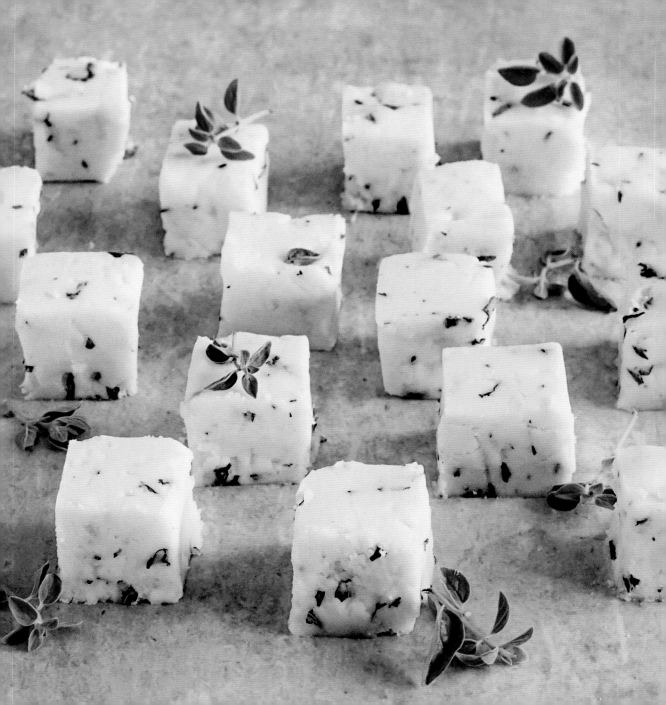

Herbal Facial Steam Tabs

½ cup (60 g) citric acid

1 cup (220 g) baking soda

2 teaspoons dried rosemary

2 teaspoons dried thyme

2 teaspoons dried mint

2 tablespoons carrier oil, such as sweet almond or sunflower

10 drops oregano essential oil

5 drops eucalyptus essential oil

30-ounce (1-L) container

Mold

4 cups (945 mL) water

I love a good steam session. It softens skin, increases circulation, and opens up pores so your favorite serums and moisturizers can penetrate the epidermis and do their thing even better. But a little tip from the esthetician: You don't have to visit the spa to enjoy the benefits of a good facial steam. These easy-to-make herbal tabs harness the antibacterial and anti-inflammatory benefits of oregano, which is used to treat both acne and rosacea.

STEP 1 / In a medium-size bowl, combine the citric acid, baking soda, and dried rosemary, thyme, and mint. Stir to combine, breaking up clumps.

STEP 2 / Decant the carrier oil of your choosing into a measuring cup, then drizzle in the oregano and eucalyptus essential oils.

STEP 3 / Pour the oil mixture into the dry ingredients, then stir until you arrive at a crumbly consistency.

STEP 4 / Use your hands to press the mixture into the wells of a mold. (A mini muffin tin or an ice cube tray works great for a batch of facial steam tabs.) Let them sit in a cool, dry place overnight.

STEP 5 / Remove the steam tabs from the mold and store them in an airtight container until you're ready to use them. (They will last up to 6 months.)

STEP 6 / When you're ready to steam, bring the water to a boil while you cleanse your face. Once boiling, transfer the water to a heat-safe bowl.

STEP 7 / Drop a steam tab into the bowl and immediately drape a towel over your head, shoulders, and the steaming water. (Or fill a sink with hot water, drop in the steam tab, and lean over the sink instead.)

STEP 8 / Keep your face about 12 to 18 inches (30–45 cm) from the steam. Enjoy for 5 to 10 minutes (and no more than 10!), then follow with a moisturizing mask or face oil. Keep your eyes closed to prevent irritation.

TIP / Oregano and eucalyptus are also great for stuffy noses and painful blocked sinuses. While your pores are soaking up the herbal benefits, take slow, deep breaths to bust up congestion.

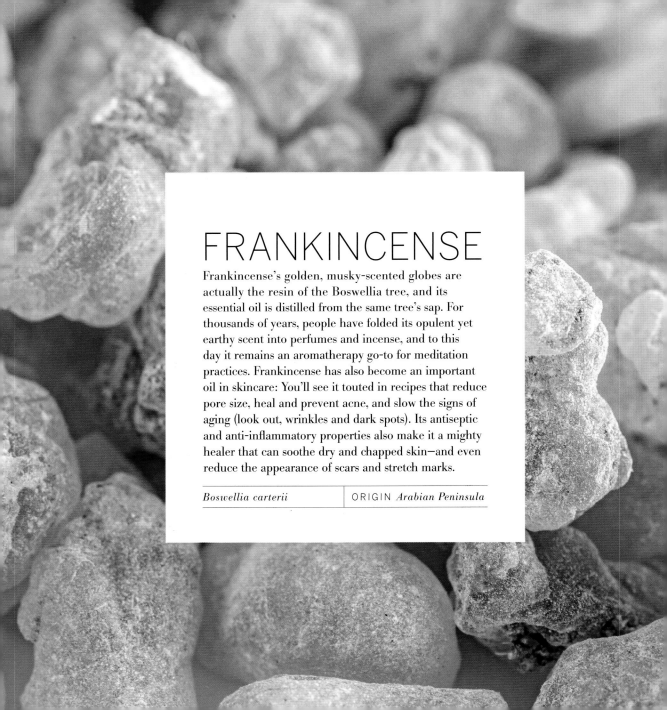

FRANKINCENSE

Frankincense's golden, musky-scented globes are actually the resin of the Boswellia tree, and its essential oil is distilled from the same tree's sap. For thousands of years, people have folded its opulent yet earthy scent into perfumes and incense, and to this day it remains an aromatherapy go-to for meditation practices. Frankincense has also become an important oil in skincare: You'll see it touted in recipes that reduce pore size, heal and prevent acne, and slow the signs of aging (look out, wrinkles and dark spots). Its antiseptic and anti-inflammatory properties also make it a mighty healer that can soothe dry and chapped skin—and even reduce the appearance of scars and stretch marks.

Boswellia carterii | ORIGIN *Arabian Peninsula*

Scar-Healing Lavender Salve

3 tablespoons lavender-infused oil (see page 16)

1 tablespoon beeswax pellets

1 tablespoon rosehip-seed oil

1 teaspoon vitamin E oil (approximately 8 capsules)

25 drops frankincense essential oil

15 drops lavender essential oil

3-ounce (90-mL) jar or three 1-ounce (30-mL) lip-balm tins

Most of us have a scar we'd rather not see every day; while inevitable, these marks from acne, burns, scrapes, and cuts can make us self-conscious. Enter frankincense and lavender essential oils, which can help reduce the appearance of scars, especially when teamed up with healing rosehip-seed and vitamin E oils.

STEP 1 / Follow the instructions on page 16 to make lavender-infused oil.

STEP 2 / Pour 2 inches (5 cm) of water into a small saucepan. Place a heat-safe glass bowl over the saucepan, then add the lavender-infused oil and beeswax.

STEP 3 / Warm over low heat until melted, then remove from the heat. Add the rosehip-seed and vitamin E oils, then the frankincense and lavender essential oils.

STEP 4 / Transfer the mixture to a jar (or several lip balm tins). Let sit until cooled completely, then cover with the lid(s).

STEP 5 / Apply a thin layer to the scar daily for 6 weeks to 2 months. Store in a cool, dry spot and use within 6 months.

Arnica-Oil Bruise Soother

¼ cup (60 mL) arnica-infused oil (see page 16)

3-ounce (90-mL) jar

12 drops frankincense essential oil

8 drops lavender essential oil

8 drops helichrysum essential oil

8 drops geranium essential oil

If you're one of those people who bruises easily, this soothing ointment is a great way to follow up an ice pack. Its powerful combination of arnica-infused oil and frankincense, lavender, helichrysum, and geranium essential oils reduces pain and can help speed the healing of those unsightly black-and-blue injuries.

STEP 1 / Infuse your preferred carrier oil with dried arnica following the instructions on page 16. (Or take a shortcut by purchasing arnica oil.)

STEP 2 / Pour the arnica oil into your jar, then drizzle in the frankincense, lavender, helichrysum, and geranium essential oils. Add the lid, then swirl to combine all the oils.

STEP 3 / Apply the oil every 2 hours until the bruise is no longer painful, swirling the bottle before each use. (Do not use arnica oil on broken skin.) Keep in a cool, dark spot and use within 6 months.

TIP / For a one-time use, just add 4 drops frankincense to 1 teaspoon arnica-infused oil.

Our poor hands really take a beating when winter hits. Even if you're good about moisturizing and wearing gloves, chances are they'll be exposed to harsh elements and dry air, as well as constant hand-washing during cold and flu season. And cracked skin doesn't just look bad—it can provide an entry point for germs. Add nourishing everyday ingredients and frankincense essential oil to your DIY manicure routine to protect your hands, give your skin a youthful glow, and reduce the appearance of dark spots.

Supersoftening Sugar Scrub

2 tablespoons sugar

2 tablespoons sweet almond oil

1 teaspoon lemon zest

1 tablespoon lemon juice

1 drop frankincense essential oil

Mix the sugar, sweet almond oil, lemon zest and juice, and frankincense essential oil in a small bowl. Gently massage a quarter-size amount into your hands using circular motions, then rinse and pat dry. You can cover and save the leftovers for up to 1 week in the fridge.

Baking Soda Hand Soak

1 cup (240 mL) warm water

1 tablespoon baking soda

1 teaspoon vegetable glycerin or carrier oil, such as grape-seed or sweet almond

5 drops frankincense essential oil

This mild nail soak will calm dry, itchy skin and replenish crucial moisture. Mix the warm water, baking soda, vegetable glycerin or oil, and frankincense essential oil in a bowl big enough to fit both hands. Soak them for 15 minutes, then gently rinse off.

Nice + Nurturing Cuticle Oil

3 drops frankincense essential oil

1 drop myrrh essential oil

⅓-ounce (10-mL) roll-on applicator

1½ teaspoons grape-seed oil

Add the frankincense and myrrh essential oils to your roll-on applicator, then measure and add the grape-seed oil. Replace the rollerball and shake to combine the oils. To apply, swipe once over each nail and gently massage into the nails and cuticles once every day. Use within 6 months.

Moisture-Boost Hand Butter

3 ounces (90 mL) coconut oil

20 drops frankincense essential oil

3-ounce (90-mL) container

Heat the coconut oil in the microwave in 10-second bursts until it melts into a liquid. Remove from the heat and drizzle in the frankincense essential oil, then mix well. Gently pour the mixture into your container. To use, rub a small amount between your hands before bed. (It helps to wear gloves overnight to seal in all that good moisture.) Store in a cool, dark spot and use within 6 months.

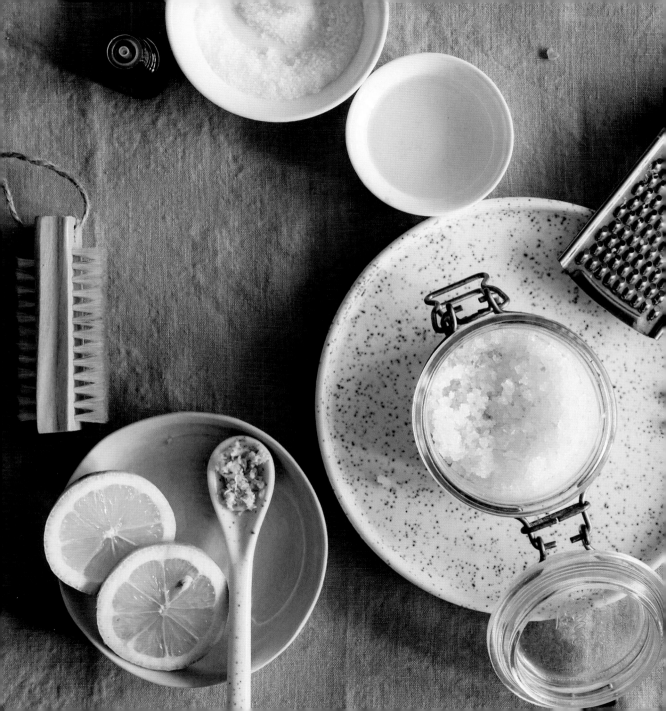

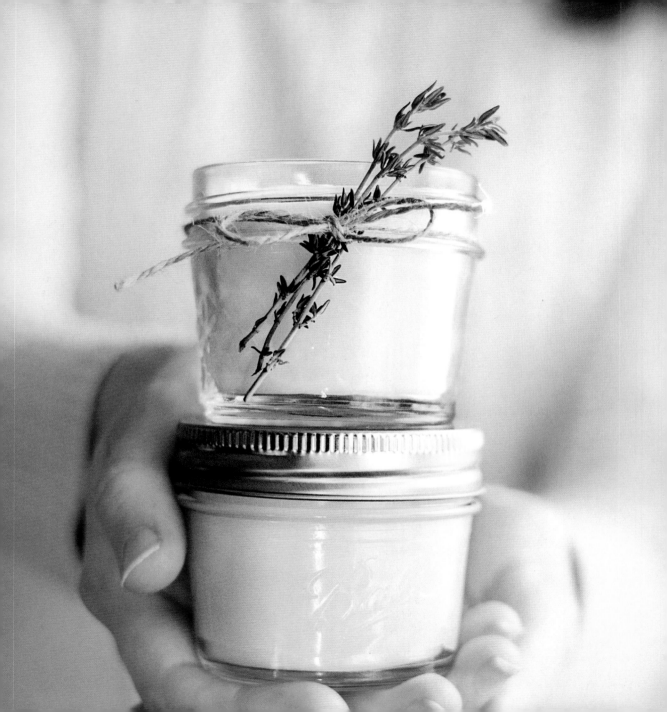

Sumptuous Slow-Cooker Candles

2 cups (475 mL) water

10 4-ounce (120-mL) mason jars with lids

4 pounds (1.8 kg) soy wax flakes

Candle dye chips (optional)

60 drops frankincense essential oil per candle

50 drops sandalwood essential oil per candle

40 drops myrrh essential oil per candle

50 drops cedarwood essential oil per candle

10 cotton wicks

Twine

Tape

Clothespin (optional)

Fresh herbs (optional)

These mason jar candles are phenomenally easy to make—just pop them in your slow cooker and let them do their thing. Frankincense essential oil gives off a cozy scent that's perfect for the holidays (or any time you want to relax by a glowing candle). Plus, these mess-free babies are made with nontoxic soy wax and 100 percent cotton wicks, so no worries about breathing dangerous fumes.

STEP 1 / Bring the water to a boil in a kettle or saucepan.

STEP 2 / Fill each mini mason jar to the top with soy wax flakes. Place the jars in your slow cooker.

STEP 3 / Pour the hot water into the slow cooker until it reaches halfway up the sides of the jars, taking care not to get water inside the jars. Place the lid on the slow cooker and set the temperature to high.

STEP 4 / After 2 hours, the wax will have melted down to half the original volume; add more wax flakes to each jar and stir. If you would like to add color to your candles, do that now by pouring in candle dye chips (available at craft stores or online).

STEP 5 / Replace the lid on the slow cooker; let sit for another hour.

STEP 6 / Once all the wax has melted, remove the jars from the slow cooker. (Be careful, they'll be hot!) Let them sit at room temperature for 10 minutes.

STEP 7 / Add 200 drops total of the frankincense, sandalwood, myrrh, and cedarwood essential oils to each jar (or for every 4 ounces/120 mL melted candle wax), then stir. These call for more essential oils than home or skincare recipes since much of the essential oil scent dissipates when mixed into the hot wax.

STEP 8 / When the wax has just started to set, insert your wicks. (You may need to use a chopstick to make a hole in the wax first.)

STEP 9 / To keep the wick upright while the wax cools, tie a piece of twine around it and secure it to one side of the jar with tape. (You can also insert the wick through the hole in the center of a wooden clothespin, then rest it on the rim of the jar while the wax sets.) Let the candles cool for several hours.

STEP 10 / Trim the wicks so that 1 inch (2.5 cm) sticks out of the candle. Add the lids and decorate the jars with twine and fresh herbs, if desired.

Slumber

At some point, we all come face to face with insomnia—we either struggle to fall asleep, or we wake up in the middle of the night and stare at the ceiling for hours. Instead of counting sheep, use the calming powers of essential oils to help you wind down and drift off to dreamland.

SLEEPYTIME BATH OIL

A warm bath calms the body and mind, setting the stage for sleep. Add the following essential oils to 2 teaspoons carrier oil (such as jojoba, sweet almond, or coconut) and pour into your warm bath.

Sweet Marjoram
4 drops

Sweet Basil
3 drops

Vetiver
3 drops

HIT-THE-HAY PILLOW SPRAY

Spritz your bed linens and the air with this dreamy mist to diffuse everyday stress and get you on your way to slumber. Add these essential oils to a spray bottle of 4 ounces (120 mL) distilled water, and mist right before you climb into bed.

Atlas Cedarwood
60 drops

Myrtle
50 drops

Spruce
40 drops

Grapefruit
25 drops

REST-EASY MASSAGE OIL

You can ease tension by applying this soothing massage oil to your upper chest, temples, and the back of your neck before bedtime. To make, dilute the following essential oils with 2 teaspoons carrier oil.

Sweet Orange
3 drops

Sweet Basil
3 drops

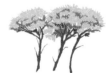

Helichrysum
4 drops

SNORE-NO-MORE DIFFUSER

If snoring keeps you or your partner awake, this blend will help keep sinuses open and restore some quiet to your sleeping space. Add these essential oils to an electric diffuser before bed and let it run all night. Adjust the volume to suit your model.

Spruce
5 drops

Tea Tree
2 drops

Eucalyptus
2 drops

Juniper Berry
1 drop

RELAXING NIGHTTIME FOOT SOAK

A simple foot soak not only soothes tired feet, it gets the entire body ready to snooze. Combine these essential oils with 1 teaspoon carrier oil—try jojoba, sweet almond, or coconut— and add to a basin of warm water. Soak your feet for at least 15 minutes.

Frankincense
3 drop

Vanilla
3 drops

Sweet Orange
3 drops

Sandalwood
1 drop

BEDSIDE-DREAM REED DIFFUSER

Your nightstand is the perfect spot for a reed diffuser. Fill yours up with a soft scent to calm worries from the day and promote sweet dreams. Add these essential oils to ¼ cup (60 mL) carrier oil in a small jar, then insert 5 or 8 reeds to disperse the scent.

Sandalwood
9 drops

Rosemary
9 drops

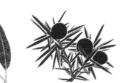

Neroli
9 drops

Geranium
9 drops

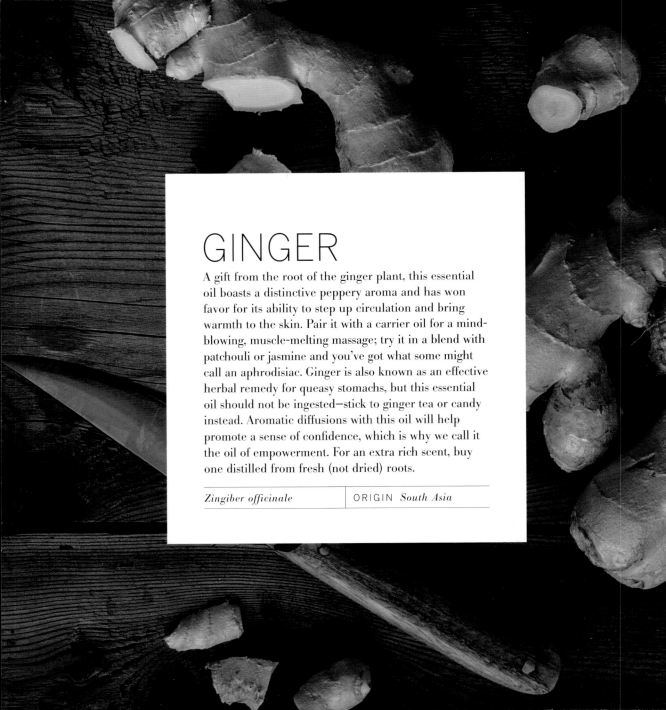

GINGER

A gift from the root of the ginger plant, this essential
oil boasts a distinctive peppery aroma and has won
favor for its ability to step up circulation and bring
warmth to the skin. Pair it with a carrier oil for a mind-
blowing, muscle-melting massage; try it in a blend with
patchouli or jasmine and you've got what some might
call an aphrodisiac. Ginger is also known as an effective
herbal remedy for queasy stomachs, but this essential
oil should not be ingested—stick to ginger tea or candy
instead. Aromatic diffusions with this oil will help
promote a sense of confidence, which is why we call it
the oil of empowerment. For an extra rich scent, buy
one distilled from fresh (not dried) roots.

Zingiber officinale | ORIGIN *South Asia*

Major-Relief Muscle Rub

2 ounces (55 g) coconut oil

1 ounce (30 mL) sweet almond or olive oil

1 teaspoon ground ginger

½ teaspoon ground cayenne

2 ounces (60 g) shea butter

½ ounce beeswax pellets (white or yellow)

6-ounce (180-mL) glass jar

20 drops ginger essential oil

15 drops eucalyptus essential oil

15 drops clary sage essential oil

5 drops peppermint essential oil

Sore muscles will usually subside on their own, but there's a lot you can do to speed up recovery—like this clever rub recipe! When capsaicin, the compound found in hot peppers and cayenne pepper, is applied to the skin, it tricks your brain into thinking it's being exposed to heat, so it releases neurotransmitters that block aches and pains. Add in some ginger for its anti-inflammatory and pain-relieving compounds, and you'll be off the couch in no time.

STEP 1 / Heat the coconut and almond or olive oils in a small glass measuring cup in 10-second blasts in the microwave until the oils are melted and combined.

STEP 2 / Add the ground ginger and cayenne, then let the mixture infuse for between 30 minutes and 1 hour.

STEP 3 / Using a cheesecloth set over a fine-mesh strainer, filter the infused oil into a heat-safe glass measuring cup with a spout. (Warm the oil again if it's too thick to strain.)

STEP 4 / Pour 2 inches (5 cm) water into a small saucepan and bring to a simmer. Add the shea butter and beeswax to the infused oil, and set the cup inside the saucepan. Heat on low until the wax and butter have melted, stirring frequently.

STEP 5 / Remove from the heat and pour the mixture into your glass jar. Add the ginger, eucalyptus, clary sage, and peppermint essential oils. (These three extra essential oils provide anti-inflammatory and

healing relief: Peppermint provides a pleasant numbing sensation, and eucalyptus oil has analgesic—aka painkilling—properties. Plus, the clary sage is both anti-inflammatory and antispasmodic.) Stir, then let cool completely before use.

STEP 6 / To apply the balm, roll a small amount between your palms to make it malleable. Rub it into sore areas in a circular motion—your skin will feel start to feel warm and tingly. Replace the lid and, when not in use, store in a cool, dark spot. Use within 6 months.

TIP / If you have sensitive skin, do a patch test on an inconspicuous area before use, and wash it off with water and soap if irritation occurs. Be careful not to get it onto mucous membranes or on broken skin. Because this balm can be a bit intense, I don't recommend it for use on children.

Ginger + Apple Cider Bath Salts

1 cup (240 g) Epsom salt

1 cup (290 g) sea salt

½ cup (110 g) baking soda

3 tablespoons ground ginger

1 tablespoon ground cinnamon

20-ounce (590-mL) container

10 drops sweet orange essential oil

6 drops ginger essential oil

4 drops patchouli essential oil

1½ cups (355 mL) apple cider vinegar

Heat things up with this decadent and warming bath soak—the ginger will make you sweat, flushing out toxins and unclogging your pores. The sea and Epsom salts provide the skin with a feast of minerals (such as calcium, potassium, and magnesium), and the apple cider vinegar helps improve dry skin and dandruff.

STEP 1 / Combine the Epsom and sea salts with the baking soda and ground ginger and cinnamon in your container. Drizzle in the sweet orange, ginger, and patchouli essential oils.

STEP 2 / Fill your tub with warm water and pour in the apple cider vinegar. Then add 3 tablespoons of the salt mixture and stir into the water until completely dissolved. (Be sure to use a dry spoon so you don't introduce moisture to the salts, which can cause them to spoil.)

STEP 3 / Step in the tub and soak for at least 30 minutes. When you're done, gently blot your skin with a towel. Use these bath salts up within 8 months.

Zesty Grapefruit Body Scrub

½ cup (125 g) sugar

1 tablespoon fresh ginger, grated

1 tablespoon grapefruit zest

¼ cup (60 mL) sweet almond oil

7 drops grapefruit essential oil

5 drops ginger essential oil

6-ounce (180-mL) jar

Take your time with this bright and spicy scrub! With both fresh ginger root and ginger essential oil, you'll get a double hit of the circulation-boosting compound zingerone. The grapefruit provides a high dose of the anti-inflammatory enzyme bromelain, which may help reduce the appearance of cellulite.

STEP 1 / Toss the sugar in a small bowl. Add the grated ginger and grapefruit zest, and stir.

STEP 2 / Pour the sweet almond oil into a measuring cup and drizzle in the grapefruit and ginger essential oils. (Ginger can overpower other scents, so start with a drop or two.)

STEP 3 / Pour the oils into the sugar mixture. Stir to thoroughly mix the ingredients, then transfer to your jar.

STEP 4 / To use, scoop out some of the mixture and, starting at your feet, scrub it all over in circular motions, avoiding sensitive areas as you move up your body. The scrubbing action will whisk away dead skin, leaving behind the nourishing almond oil. Refrigerate and use within 7 days.

TIP / Use this scrub in the shower, or put down a towel and apply it before hopping in the ginger and apple cider bath above.

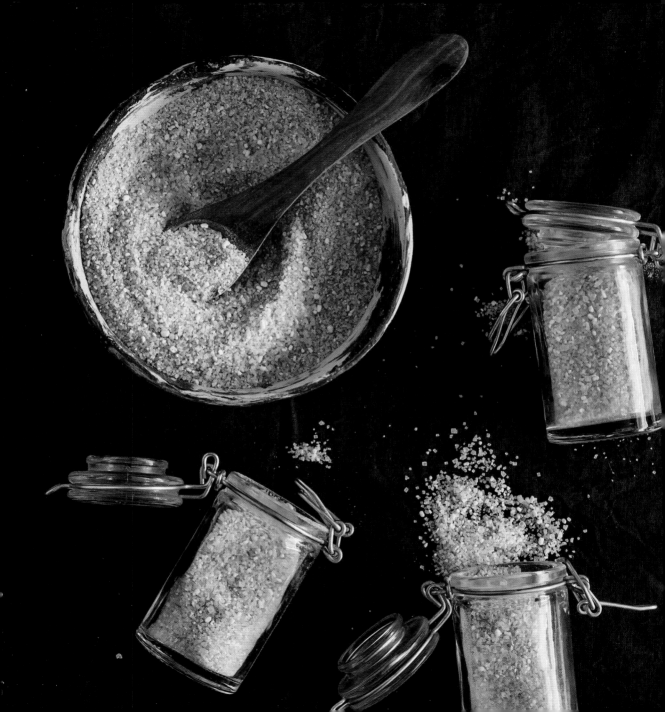

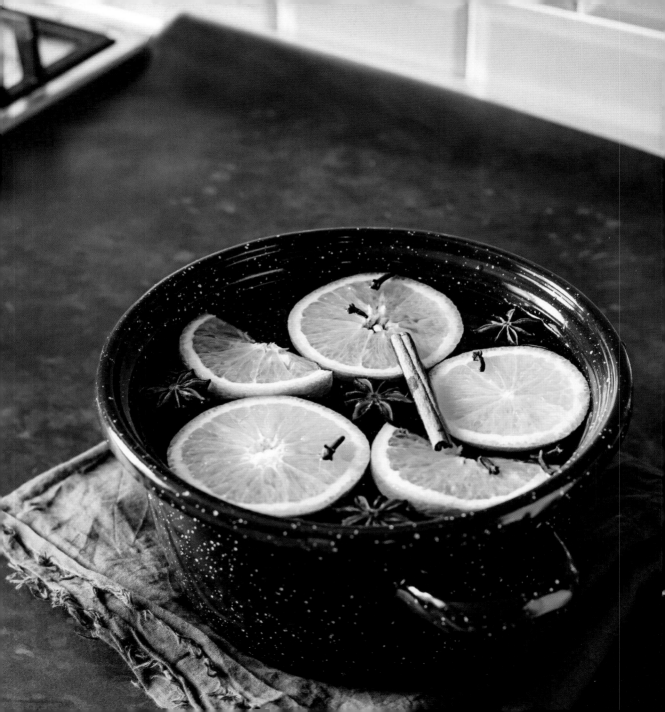

Purifying Orange-Spice Pot Simmer

25 drops sweet orange essential oil

14 drops ginger essential oil

7 drops nutmeg or allspice essential oil

4 drops cinnamon bark essential oil

2-mL dark glass bottle

1 quart (945 mL) water

1 fresh orange, sliced

5 whole cloves

1 cinnamon stick

3 whole star anise

If the world knew how effective natural ingredients were at keeping the air clean, room freshener sales would definitely take a hit. Pot simmers are just about the easiest way to purify and sweeten the air, and they cost just pennies to make. Simply mix together your favorite essential oils (plus a few fragrant dried herbs and spices), then add water and heat. This citrus-ginger variation is an instant way to brighten and invigorate your whole household.

STEP 1 / Drizzle the sweet orange, ginger, nutmeg or allspice, and cinnamon bark essential oils into your bottle. Add the cap and mix the oils well by rolling it between your hands.

STEP 2 / Fill a large pot with the water and bring to a simmer. Add 5 drops of the essential oil blend, then toss in the nutmeg or allspice, fresh orange slices, whole cloves, cinnamon stick, and star anise.

STEP 3 / To make your home smell warm and inviting, let simmer for 15 to 20 minutes. (You can keep it going even longer—just add more water as needed.) This blend can be used to make approximately 10 pot simmers; use within 1 year.

STEP 4 / Spice rack looking bare these days? You can diffuse the oil blend on its own in a mini crockpot set to low or in your electric diffuser.

MORE GREAT POT SIMMERS

The best thing about pot simmers? They're endlessly customizable. Build one around your favorite essential oils or just to use up what's hogging space in your cabinet. Here are a few ideas.

SANDALWOOD-VANILLA 1 vanilla bean, 2 drops each sandalwood and vanilla, and 1 drop clove bud.

CITRUS-FIR 3 to 4 dried orange slices, 1 to 2 tablespoons dried lemon peel, 2 drops each sweet orange and fir, and 1 drop lemon.

SPICED COFFEE ¼ cup (25 g) whole roasted coffee beans, 2 drops sweet orange, and 1 drop each cinnamon, clove bud, and vanilla.

CINNAMON-GRAPEFRUIT 1 stick cinnamon, 1 grapefruit peel, 1 shake ground nutmeg or allspice, 3 drops grapefruit, and 1 drop each cinnamon and clove bud.

PEPPERMINT-ROSEMARY 1 large sprig fresh rosemary, 3 drops peppermint, 2 drops rosemary, and 1 drop eucalyptus.

CRAN-APPLE SPICE ¼ cup (30 g) dried cranberries, ¼ cup (30 g) dried apple rings, 2 drops each cardamom and cinnamon, and 1 drop each ginger and clove bud.

FRANKINCENSE-JUNIPER 1 tablespoon dried juniper berries, 3 drops each frankincense and fir, and 2 drops each juniper and bergamot.

TEA TREE

Long used by indigenous Australians to treat colds
and wounds, tea tree essential oil is known for its
antifungal, antiseptic, antibiotic, and skin-soothing
powers—and for its bright medicinal scent. It's widely
used as a topical fix for skin problems including acne,
burns, dandruff, and athlete's foot; scientists are even
exploring it as a treatment for staph, vaginal infections,
and herpes. Inhaling tea tree essential oil—by diffusing
it or adding it to a bath—can open up sinuses and ease
coughing. Beyond skincare and colds, this stuff is a
great disinfectant for surfaces in your home, and it can
even act as a spot treatment for small areas of mold.

Melaleuca alternifolia | ORIGIN *Oceania*

DIY Antibiotic Salve

½ cup (120 mL) olive oil
½ cup (100 g) coconut oil
⅓ cup (25 g) dried calendula
⅓ cup (25 g) dried lavender
4 tablespoons beeswax pellets
1 tablespoon honey
50 drops tea tree essential oil
25 drops lavender essential oil
12-ounce (355-mL) jar

Cuts, scrapes, burns, and other minor skin wounds are inevitable, especially if you have kiddos in the house (or even if you're just sort of a clumsy adult—no shame in that). This all-natural DIY combo of tea tree essential oil, calendula, lavender, and honey—along with the moisturizing ingredients coconut and olive oil—will help your skin heal. It's not just for injuries, either: Feel free to slather it on chapped hands or dry feet when lotion just won't cut it.

STEP 1 / Bring 2 inches (5 cm) of water to boil in a small saucepan. Reduce the heat to low.

STEP 2 / Combine the olive and coconut oils in a heat-safe glass bowl and place it over the saucepan. Stir until the coconut oil has melted and combined with the olive oil.

STEP 3 / Add in the dried calendula and lavender. Simmer on low heat for at least 30 minutes. Pour more water into the saucepan, as needed.

STEP 4 / Filter the oil mixture through a fine-mesh strainer. Discard the herbs.

STEP 5 / Wipe the glass bowl clean and pour the strained oil mixture back into it. Place the bowl once again inside the saucepan, then add in the beeswax pellets and honey. Stir over low heat until the mixture has melted.

STEP 6 / Remove from the heat and drizzle in the tea tree and lavender essential oils, stirring to combine.

STEP 7 / Pour the mixture into your jar and allow it to cool and set for about 20 minutes. Add the lid.

STEP 8 / To administer, use a cotton swab to apply the salve to clean skin twice a day, then cover with a fresh adhesive bandage. Store in a cool, dark place and use within 1 year.

At once calming and invigorating, tea tree essential oil is a great choice for just about any skin type, and a little goes a long way. Some studies have shown that a 5 percent solution works just as well as 5 percent benzoyl peroxide on severe acne—and it does so without leaving your skin flaky and zapped of natural moisture like the store-bought stuff does. Even if you're not breakout-prone, tea tree essential oil makes a great toner; just pair it with a nongreasy carrier oil.

Zit-Curing Face Mask

4 tablespoons aloe vera gel

½ peeled cucumber, roughly chopped

3 drops tea tree essential oil

Use a blender to combine the aloe vera gel and cucumber into a smooth paste. Transfer the mixture to a small bowl and stir in the tea tree essential oil. Apply the mixture to your face with your fingertips or a facial brush, and leave it on for 10 to 15 minutes. Rinse with warm water and follow up with moisturizer.

Garlic + Tea Tree Spot Treatment

½ clove fresh garlic, finely minced

½ teaspoon jojoba oil

2 drops tea tree essential oil

Mix the minced garlic and jojoba oil in a small bowl, then stir in the tea tree essential oil. Apply the mixture to acne spots or pimples with a clean finger or cotton swab. Leave the spot treatment on overnight and wash it off in the morning. This mixture can be stored in the refrigerator for a few days, but fresh is best for potency, so make it in small batches as needed.

Anti-Acne Roll-On

⅓-ounce (10-mL) roll-on applicator

⅓ ounce (10 mL) carrier oil, such as jojoba, hempseed, or grape-seed

12 drops tea tree essential oil

Fill the roll-on applicator almost to the top with your choice of carrier oil, then add the tea tree essential oil. Pop the rollerball back into the applicator tube and roll it between your hands to gently mix the oils together. To fight a breakout, roll a thin layer onto your skin 1 or 2 times per day. Use within 6 months.

Hit Refresh Basil Facial Steam

3 cups (710 mL) water

6 fresh basil leaves

3 drops tea tree essential oil

Bring the water to a boil while you wash your face. Carefully transfer the water to a heat-safe bowl and add the basil leaves and tea tree essential oil. Immediately drape a large towel over your head, shoulders, and the bowl, keeping your face about 10 to 18 inches (25–46 cm) from the water's surface. Enjoy the steam for 5 to 10 minutes, then follow with a mask, serum, or moisturizer while your skin is still damp.

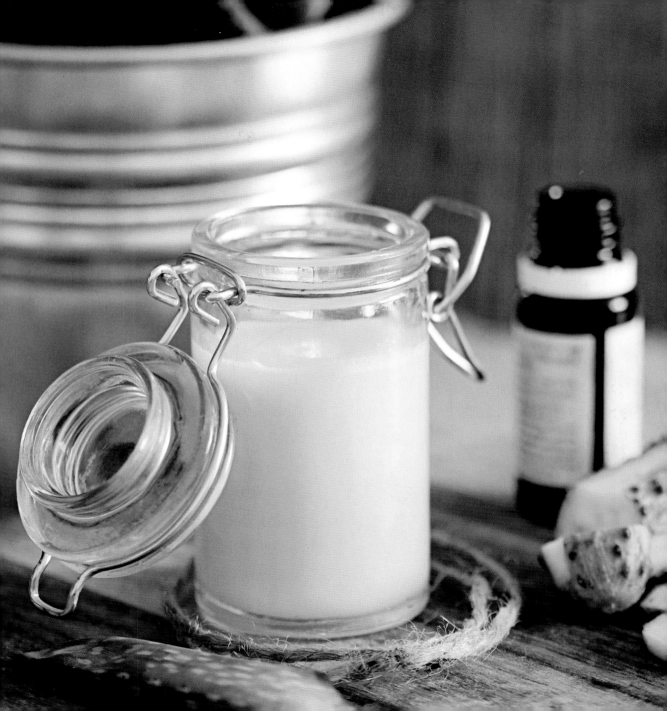

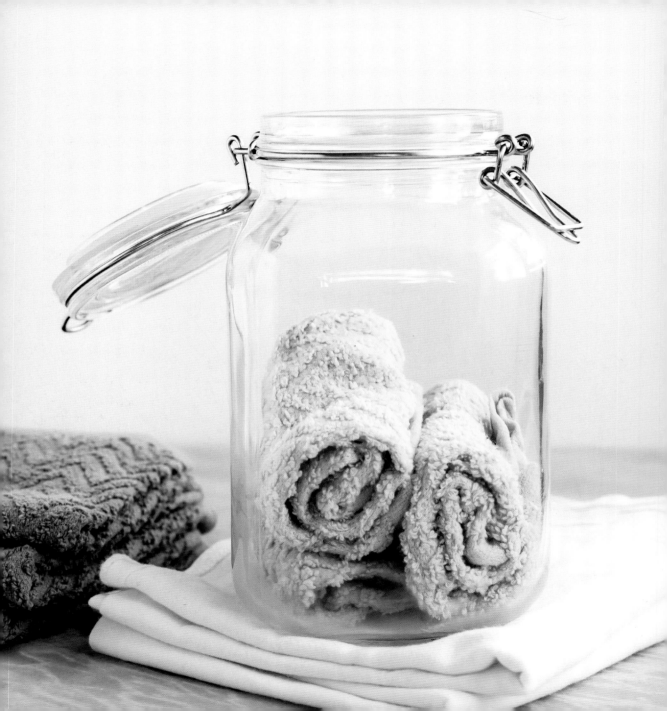

Reusable Disinfectant Wipes

3 teaspoons natural liquid dish soap

50 to 75 drops tea tree essential oil

3 cups (710 mL) distilled white vinegar

Reusable cloths, such as washcloths, old T-shirts cut into squares, or socks cut into strips

3-quart (3-L) glass jar

How did we ever keep our homes clean before the invention of disinfectant wipes? With a little creativity, you can make your own ecofriendly, all-natural, reusable version of these handy squares—with a dose of tea tree essential oil to make them antimicrobial. You'll never go back to the disposable kind.

STEP 1 / Combine the liquid dish soap, tea tree essential oil, and white vinegar in a large bowl. Stir well.

STEP 2 / Toss your old cloths into the bowl and allow them to soak up your soapy solution, then squeeze out any excess liquid.

STEP 3 / Roll up the wipes and store them in the large glass jar for speedy, no-fuss cleaning of just about every surface. Once used, wash and repeat; use within 1 year.

TIP / You can also store the wipes and solution separately, then quickly wet the wipes when you need them.

Game-Changing Nontoxic Tub Scrub

½ cup (110 g) baking soda

½ cup (140 g) washing soda

¼ cup (70 g) salt

½ cup (120 mL) unscented liquid castile soap

25 drops tea tree essential oil

2 tablespoons hydrogen peroxide (optional)

Scrubbing the tub is a less than delightful task. The soap scum, odd angles, and sheer size of the project can be daunting, so let this awesome scrub help you out! Baking soda and salt make a gritty base for the bleaching power of hydrogen peroxide, while the castile soap and tea tree essential oil redefine "clean."

STEP 1 / Combine the baking soda, washing soda, and salt in a small bowl. (What's washing soda? Sometimes called laundry soda or soda crystals, washing soda is a high-alkaline powder that helps make your regular soaps and detergent more effective, particularly in hard water areas.)

STEP 2 / Slowly add the unscented liquid castile soap. Stir until the mixture turns into a fine paste.

STEP 3 / Drizzle in the tea tree essential oil and mix thoroughly. If you're using the hydrogen peroxide to introduce some extra whitening power, now's the time to add it.

STEP 4 / Whenever you're ready to tackle the tub, just scoop a little out and scrub away with your dry sponge. Use within 6 months.

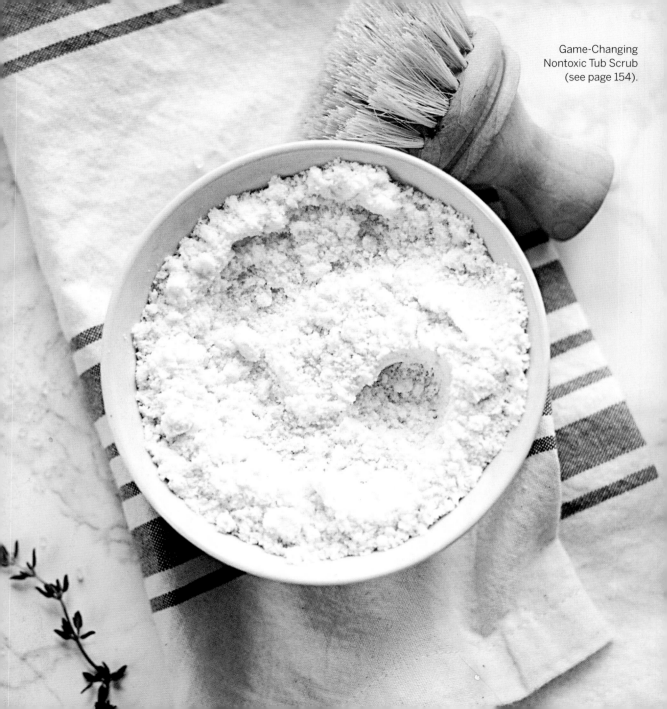

Game-Changing
Nontoxic Tub Scrub
(see page 154).

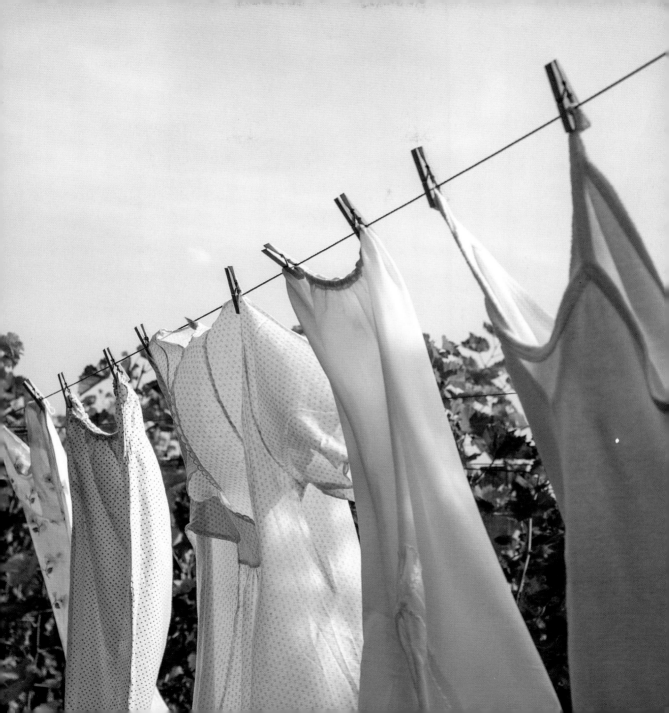

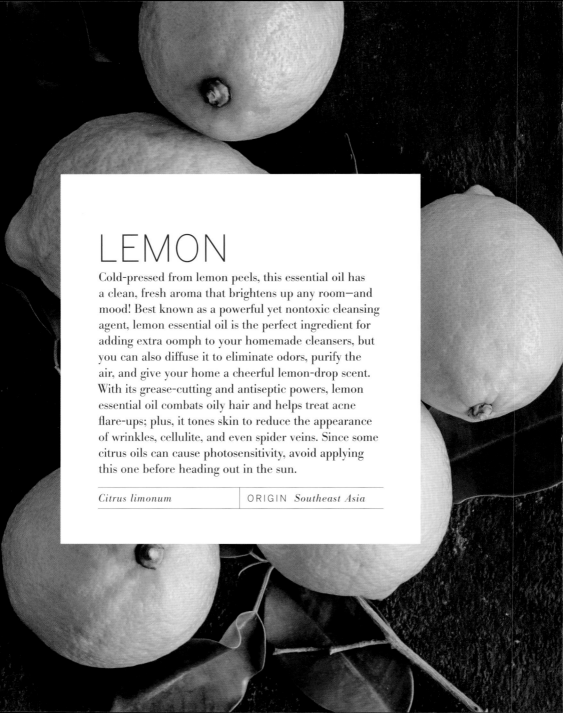

LEMON

Cold-pressed from lemon peels, this essential oil has a clean, fresh aroma that brightens up any room—and mood! Best known as a powerful yet nontoxic cleansing agent, lemon essential oil is the perfect ingredient for adding extra oomph to your homemade cleansers, but you can also diffuse it to eliminate odors, purify the air, and give your home a cheerful lemon-drop scent. With its grease-cutting and antiseptic powers, lemon essential oil combats oily hair and helps treat acne flare-ups; plus, it tones skin to reduce the appearance of wrinkles, cellulite, and even spider veins. Since some citrus oils can cause photosensitivity, avoid applying this one before heading out in the sun.

Citrus limonum | ORIGIN *Southeast Asia*

Morning Jump-Start Shower Tablets

1 cup (220 g) baking soda
1 cup (130 g) cornstarch
Zest of 1 lemon
Zest of 1 lime
¼ cup (60 mL) water
1 teaspoon lemon essential oil
30 drops grapefruit essential oil
30 drops lime essential oil
Mold
30-ounce (1-L) jar

If you're not a morning person, these energizing shower melts are just the incentive you need to get out of bed. This sunny blend of lemon, lime, and grapefruit will scent your whole bathroom and help you wake up happy. Shower tablets are supereasy and inexpensive to make—you only need baking soda, cornstarch, and water. I've added energizing, uplifting citrus to clear the mind, improve positivity, and support creativity.

STEP 1 / Add the baking soda, cornstarch, and lemon and lime zest to a large mixing bowl. Stir until well blended.

STEP 2 / Add the water to make a paste that holds together in clumps without being soupy or runny. Add ½ teaspoon lemon essential oil, then drizzle in the entire allotment of the grapefruit and lime essential oils.

STEP 3 / Dollop 1 to 2 tablespoons of the mixture into the wells of a small mold—a cupcake pan will do the trick. (Using cupcake liners or silicone molds will make it easier to remove the disks later.)

STEP 4 / Preheat the oven to 350°F (177°C) and bake the mixture for 15 to 20 minutes. Remove and let cool completely. Don't worry if the tablets look a little moist—they'll continue drying as they cool.

STEP 5 / Sprinkle the tablets with the remaining ½ teaspoon lemon essential oil. Allow it to soak in.

STEP 6 / To use, place one tablet on the bottom of the shower and run hot water over it, then hop in. (You can also add one to your bathwater.)

STEP 7 / Store the tablets in a large jar for up to 6 months.

Wipe-the-Day-Away Eye Makeup Remover

2 tablespoons witch hazel

2 tablespoons jojoba oil

1 tablespoon aloe vera gel

3-ounce (90-mL) bottle

2 drops lemon essential oil

While natural cleansers are an upgrade over nonorganic versions, they don't remove mascara and eye makeup quite as well—and sleeping in that gunk can cause zits and even premature aging. This daily remedy goes easy on the eyes with witch hazel, jojoba oil, and aloe vera, plus lemon essential oil to cut grease.

STEP 1 / Combine the witch hazel, jojoba oil, and aloe vera gel in a small measuring cup. (Make sure your aloe vera gel is natural—not the goopy green gel you find in drugstores.)

STEP 2 / Pour the mixture into your bottle. Drizzle in the lemon essential oil, then replace the bottle's cap and swirl to mix the ingredients.

STEP 3 / Before each use, agitate the liquid to recombine. Then dispense a small amount onto a cotton pad, close your eyes, and gently wipe over the eye area. Don't tug or pull on the delicate eye area—it's a big no-no if you want to avoid wrinkles (and who doesn't?!). Be sure to use within 3 months, and avoid introducing water to the mixture.

All-Natural Makeup Brush Cleaner

¼ cup (60 mL) unscented liquid castile soap

2 tablespoons olive oil

3-ounce (90-mL) bottle

5 drops lemon essential oil

¼ cup (60 mL) witch hazel

Think of your makeup brushes like paintbrushes: You wouldn't start a new masterpiece with dried-up pigment on your brushes—especially if you've invested in nice ones. Here's a simple, natural makeup brush cleaner that'll help keep your tools (and your pores) clear of old makeup gunk.

STEP 1 / Combine the liquid castile soap and olive oil in your bottle. (If it's a different size, adjust the volume— just keep the 2:1 soap-to-oil ratio.)

STEP 2 / Drizzle in the lemon essential oil, replace the lid, and swirl to combine.

STEP 3 / Before each use, first agitate the bottle to recombine the ingredients. Pour some of the makeup cleaner into a small dish. Dip your

brush into the mixture and coat the bristles, then swish the brush back and forth in the palm of your hand. Get some good suds going!

STEP 4 / Rinse the brush until the water runs clean. Finish by spritzing it with a bottle of witch hazel to kill any bacteria. Lay the brushes flat to dry.

STEP 5 / Repeat as often as desired (after each use or daily, but at least weekly). Use within 1 year.

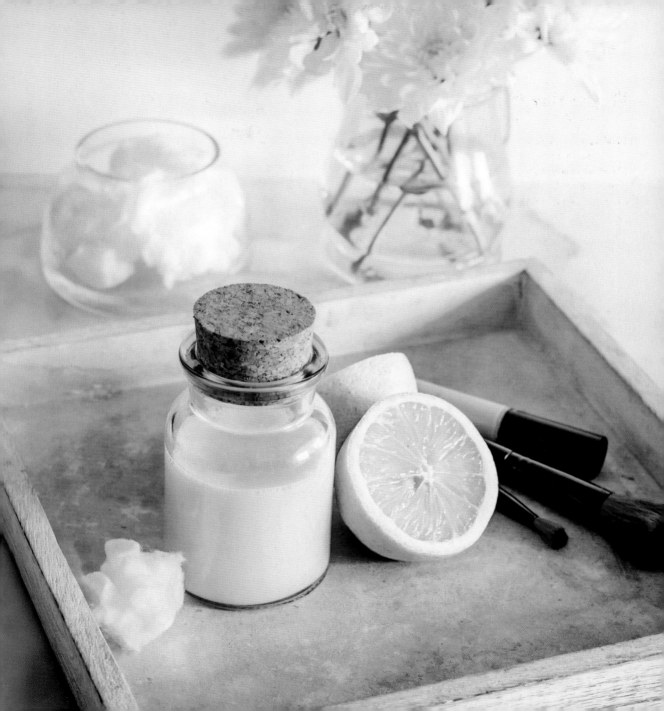

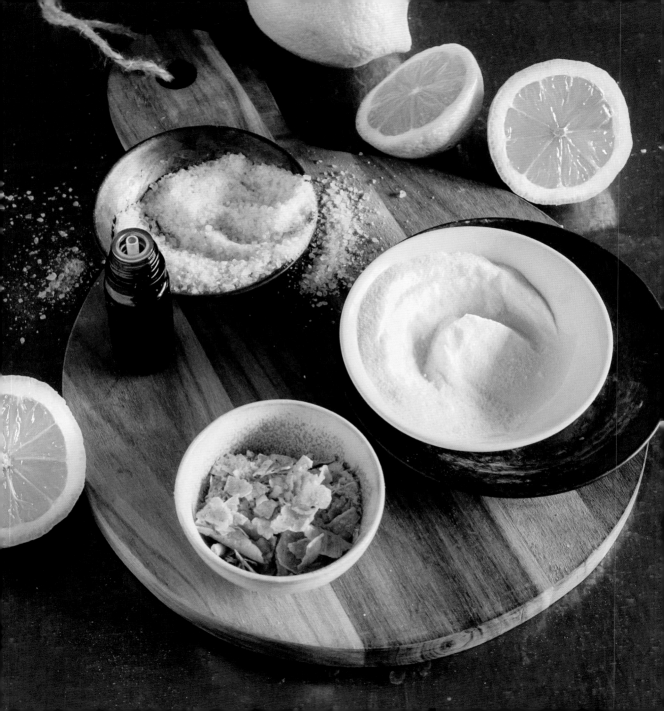

Beloved for its light, clean, and crisp citrus scent, lemon essential oil is a powerhouse in homemade cleaning recipes. Combined with a few simple ingredients—think salt, baking soda, and liquid castile soap—you can render your home spotless without the toxic chemicals found in store-bought cleaners. Naturally antibacterial and antiseptic, lemon essential oil is especially awesome in the kitchen, where it can degrease stubborn food stuck to dishes as well as freshen the air.

Citrus Cutting Board Scrub

¼ cup (10 g) soap flakes

½ cup (145 g) coarse salt

½ cup (110 g) baking soda

10 drops lemon essential oil

12-ounce (355-mL) jar

½ lemon (optional)

Combine the soap flakes, coarse salt, and baking soda in a mixing bowl. Drizzle in the lemon essential oil and stir, then transfer to your jar. To use, sprinkle on cutting boards and counters—or on dirty pots and pans—and wipe clean. For tough jobs, apply the scrub with the cut side of a lemon half—it'll disinfect and kill odors too.

Simple Fridge Deodorizer

20 drops lemon essential oil

16-ounce (455-g) box baking soda

Stir the lemon essential oil into your box of baking soda. Place the open box in the back of your fridge to absorb odors and make it smell fresh and clean. To give it a burst of freshness, periodically stir to release the scent from the essential oils. Add more if the scent starts to dissipate. Replace with fresh baking soda and essential oils every 3 to 4 months.

Miraculous Microwave Cleaner

2 cups (475 mL) water

1 lemon, halved

5 drops lemon essential oil

Pour the water into a microwave-safe glass bowl, then add the lemon halves and essential oil. Cook on high for 3 minutes. The hot, lemony steam will coat the inside of the microwave, allowing for easy removal of debris and food remnants. Simply wipe with a damp cloth to erase all that ickiness!

Lemon Multipurpose Spray

2 cups (475 mL) water

2 tablespoons unscented liquid castile soap

1 teaspoon borax

½ teaspoon washing soda

20 drops lemon essential oil

16-ounce (475-mL) spray bottle

Combine the water, unscented liquid castile soap, borax, washing soda, and lemon essential oil in your spray bottle and shake well. Spray on fridges, stoves, and countertops to cut through greasy stains. For stuck-on grime, wait 5 minutes after spraying before wiping the surface down with a scrub sponge.

Immunity

When cold and flu season hit, turn to an arsenal of powerful antiviral and antibacterial essential oils to help prevent illness and improve recovery. Note that some of these essential oils are potential skin irritants, so always dilute according to the brand instructions and test before topical use.

GERM-SLAYING HAND SANITIZER

Cleanliness is your first line of defense against annoying colds. Mix these essential oils with 1 tablespoon aloe vera gel in a 1-ounce (30-mL) spray bottle, then top it off with witch hazel. Shake and spritz on your hands to kill germs as well as clear your mind.

Tea Tree
4 drops

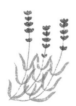

Lavender
4 drops

Geranium
2 drops

Rosemary
2 drops

KID-FRIENDLY HAND SOAP

Replace harsh antibacterial soaps with this gentle version, which is safe to use with children—who we all know are the ultimate germ carriers! In an 8-ounce (240-mL) pump bottle, add these essential oils and 3 tablespoons unscented liquid castile soap, then fill it up with distilled water.

Atlas Cedarwood
2 drops

Lemon
3 drops

Tea Tree
4 drops

MIGHTY DISINFECTING SPRAY

In a spray bottle, add 20 drops of this essential oil blend for every 1 ounce (30 mL) hydrogen peroxide. To use, first clean your home's surfaces with vinegar, then follow up with this spritz to kill even more germs. Just don't mix hydrogen and vinegar together in the same bottle!

Cinnamon Leaf
6 drops

Eucalyptus
8 drops

Lemon
6 drops

FEEL-BETTER-SOON BATH SOAK

When your body is trying to fight off flu symptoms, not much feels better than a long soak in a warm bath—especially one that's been dosed with restorative essential oils. Combine the following oils with 1 tablespoon carrier oil and swirl into your bathwater.

Roman
Chamomile
2 drops

Melissa
2 drops

Frankincense
1 drop

TRAVEL-SICKNESS INHALER

Don't let a sensitive stomach put up a road block in your roadtrip! If you get motion sick when you're in a car or on a boat or a plane, add these essential oils to a tissue or handkerchief. Keep it in your pocket and pull it out to inhale as needed.

Ginger
2 drops

Sweet Orange
2 drops

Roman
Chamomile
2 drops

IMMUNE-SUPPORT DIFFUSION

We all get tired and burned out—which leaves the door open for pesky bacteria looking to set up camp in a weaken host body. Add a few drops of this uplifting blend to an electric diffuser to keep germs at bay. Adjust the volume per your diffuser model's instructions.

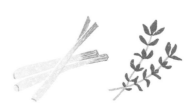

Lemongrass
3 drops

Thyme
3 drops

Clove Bud
3 drops

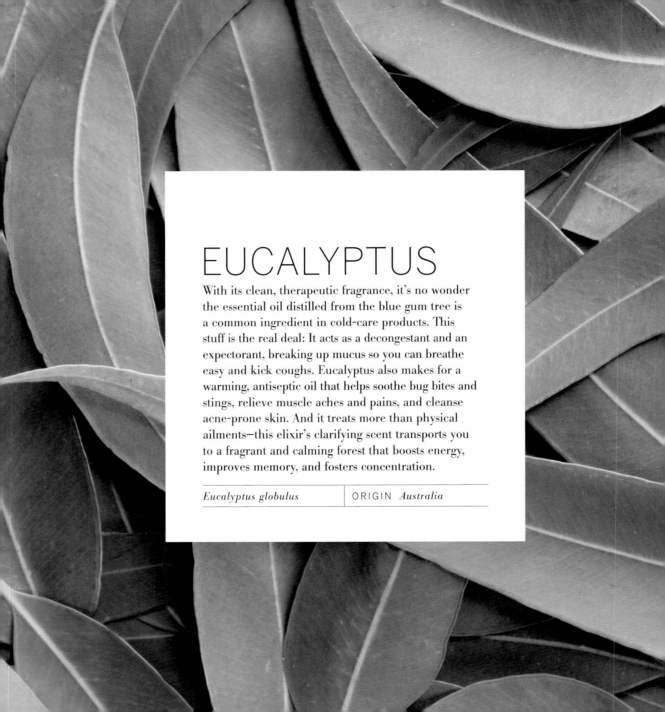

EUCALYPTUS

With its clean, therapeutic fragrance, it's no wonder the essential oil distilled from the blue gum tree is a common ingredient in cold-care products. This stuff is the real deal: It acts as a decongestant and an expectorant, breaking up mucus so you can breathe easy and kick coughs. Eucalyptus also makes for a warming, antiseptic oil that helps soothe bug bites and stings, relieve muscle aches and pains, and cleanse acne-prone skin. And it treats more than physical ailments—this elixir's clarifying scent transports you to a fragrant and calming forest that boosts energy, improves memory, and fosters concentration.

| *Eucalyptus globulus* | ORIGIN *Australia* |

Wake-Me-Up Shower Scrub

3 tablespoons whole almonds

4 tablespoons old-fashioned oats

½ cup (120 mL) unscented liquid castile soap

2 tablespoons sweet almond oil

24 drops eucalyptus essential oil

6-ounce (180-mL) squeeze or pump bottle

If you count on a shower to get you going in the a.m., why not dose it with aromatherapy for a great start to your day? Eucalyptus's restorative scent clears a still-sleepy brain, and it stimulates circulation to get the blood moving to tired limbs. When combined with exfoliating almonds and oats, you get a gentle cleanser that sloughs off dead skin and tones tough oily or acne-prone patches.

STEP 1 / Combine the almonds and old-fashioned oats in a food processor. Pulse into a medium-fine meal—perfect for some gentle exfoliation.

STEP 2 / In a mixing bowl, combine the ground meal with the unscented liquid castile soap, sweet almond oil, and eucalyptus essential oil. Stir gently to avoid creating bubbles.

STEP 3 / Transfer the mixture to your squeeze or pump bottle.

STEP 4 / To use in the shower, simply squeeze out a small amount onto your washcloth or shower pouf, then scrub all over and rinse. Use within 1 month.

Charcoal Blackhead-Busting Mask

2 tablespoons unscented liquid castile soap

1 tablespoon apricot kernel oil

2 tablespoons finely ground brown or white rice flour

1 tablespoon baking soda

2 teaspoons activated charcoal

1 drop eucalyptus essential oil

4-ounce (120-mL) airtight container

Pores plugged up with sebum, makeup, and dead skin cells turn dark when they open up to the air—hence the gross "blackhead" monicker. Beat them back with activated charcoal (known for removing impurities from the skin) and antibacterial eucalyptus essential oil, plus exfoliating baking soda and flour.

STEP 1 / In a small bowl, mix the unscented liquid castile soap and apricot kernel oil. Add the rice flour, baking soda, and activated charcoal.

STEP 2 / Drizzle in the eucalyptus essential oil. Stir until the mixture is creamy, then transfer to a container.

STEP 3 / To use as a scrub, splash your face with warm water and apply 1 to 2 teaspoons of the mixture to your face with your fingertips, scrubbing in small, circular motions while avoiding the eye area. To use as a mask, let it sit for a few minutes for extra oil-absorbing benefits. Rinse with warm water and pat dry.

STEP 4 / Store in a cool, dry place and use within 3 months. (If the scrub becomes dry, add a little water or almond oil and stir to make it rich and buttery again.)

DIY Vapor Chest Rub

¼ cup (50 g) coconut oil

1 tablespoon beeswax

10 drops eucalyptus essential oil

8 drops rosemary essential oil

5 drops peppermint
essential oil

13 drops cypress essential oil

3-ounce (90-mL) glass jar

Fighting off a cold requires lots of rest—which is hard when you're up all night coughing. Thanks to congestion-busting eucalyptus and menthol-rich peppermint essential oils, this easy DIY remedy mimics the effects of Vicks, clearing airways and smoothing over coughs so you can sleep and get well.

STEP 1 / Mix the coconut oil and beeswax in a heat-safe glass bowl.

STEP 2 / Pour 2 inches (5 cm) of water into a saucepan. Place the bowl over the saucepan; heat over low to melt the oil and beeswax together.

STEP 3 / Remove the bowl from the heat and let cool. Stir in the eucalyptus, rosemary, peppermint, and cypress essential oils.

STEP 4 / Pour the mixture into the jar; let it cool to room temperature.

STEP 5 / Massage the rub into your chest, back, and feet. Store covered with a lid and use within 6 months.

TIP / Eucalyptus, rosemary, and peppermint essential oils are not recommended for use with young children. Instead, you can make this recipe with just cypress essential oil, using 3 drops for ages 2 to 6 (a 0.25 percent dilution) or 12 drops for ages 6 to 10 (a 1 percent dilution).

Cold Season Survival Bath

2 cups (440 g) baking soda

1 cup (290 g) sea salt

1 cup (240 g) Epsom salt

3 tablespoons grape-seed oil

10 drops eucalyptus essential oil

20 drops lemon essential oil

8 drops tea tree essential oil

12 drops helichrysum
essential oil

32-ounce (950-mL) jar

Adding stimulating and rejuvenating eucalyptus essential oil to this simple detox bath can help open up congested sinuses and get a cough under control. Make this your go-to bath any time you feel a cold coming on! Or use it weekly as a purifying, stress-relieving ritual.

STEP 1 / In a mixing bowl, combine the baking soda with the sea and Epsom salts. Stir until well combined.

STEP 2 / Sprinkle the mixture with grape-seed oil and eucalyptus, lemon, tea tree, and helichrysum essential oils. Whisk until smoothly mixed.

STEP 3 / Scoop the bath mixture into your jar and replace the lid. Store and use within 6 months.

STEP 4 / To use, run a hot bath and dissolve ½ cup (30 g) of the salts. Soak for 30 minutes to 1 hour to help open up your lungs and ease coughs.

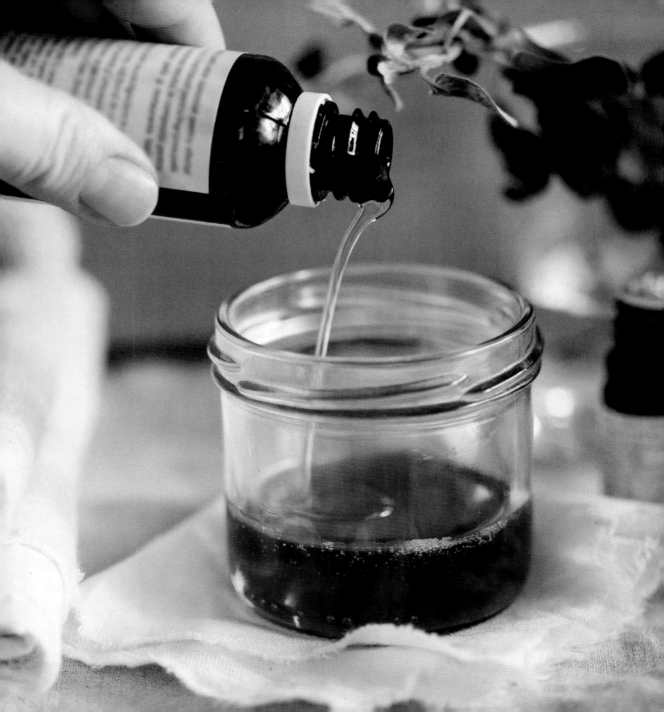

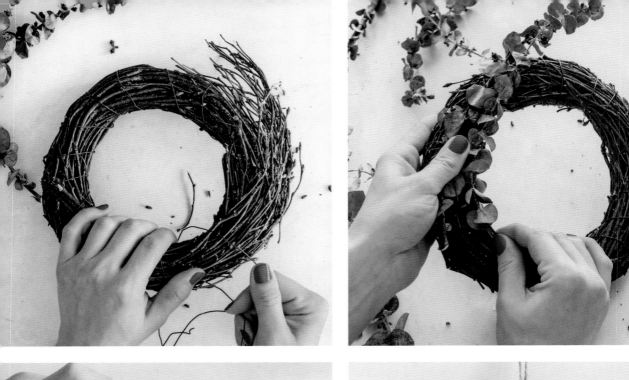

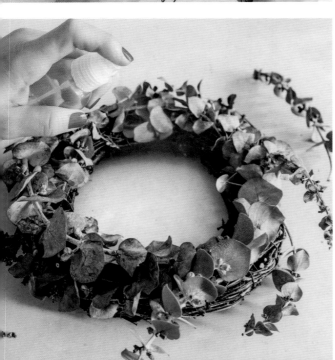

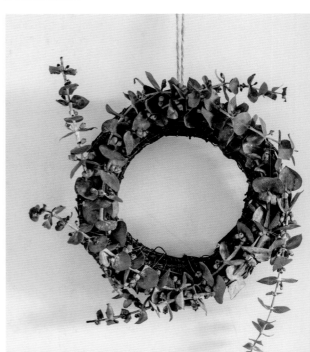

Fresh + Friendly Eucalyptus Wreath

10 to 12 long pieces of grapevine

Wire cutters

Eucalyptus stems

Floral wire

Decorative ribbon (optional)

10 drops eucalyptus essential oil

1-ounce (30-mL) spray bottle

1 ounce (30 mL) distilled water

Give me a bouquet of these pretty green stems over flowers any day! This wreath makes a stylish, natural, and year-round decoration, and it adds wonderful fragrance to your home—the trick is to keep it going by adding a few drops of eucalyptus essential oil as the wreath dries. It's particularly lovely if you hang it in the bathroom, where steam helps release its eucalyptus aroma. If you don't think of yourself as crafty, take heart: This project is meant to look a bit wild.

STEP 1 / Bundle the grapevine pieces together and coil them into a 14-inch (36-cm) circle, overlapping the ends by 1 inch (2.5 cm) or so and securing with floral wire. (You can also use a store-bought wreath form—look for them in craft outlets.)

STEP 2 / Use the wire cutters to trim the eucalyptus stems into 6- to 8-inch (15–20-cm) sprigs. (Longer stems are better.) Cut the ends on a diagonal and remove the leaves to expose 1 inch (2.5 cm) of stem at the bottom of each sprig.

STEP 3 / Begin wrapping the longer, heartier sprigs around the wreath form. Insert the stems into the wreath, evenly distributing them in a clockwise direction around the circle.

STEP 4 / Fill in any gaps with smaller eucalyptus sprigs and any additional desired greenery or flowers. (Sage, lavender, and bay leaves would all work well.) Secure the eucalyptus and any other greenery with more floral wire.

STEP 5 / If you're using a decorative ribbon, tie it to the wreath. Your wreath is ready to hang!

STEP 6 / Drizzle 10 drops eucalyptus essential oil into a spray bottle, then fill with the distilled water. Spritz the wreath regularly to help it retain its fragrance, extending the life of this beautiful home decor.

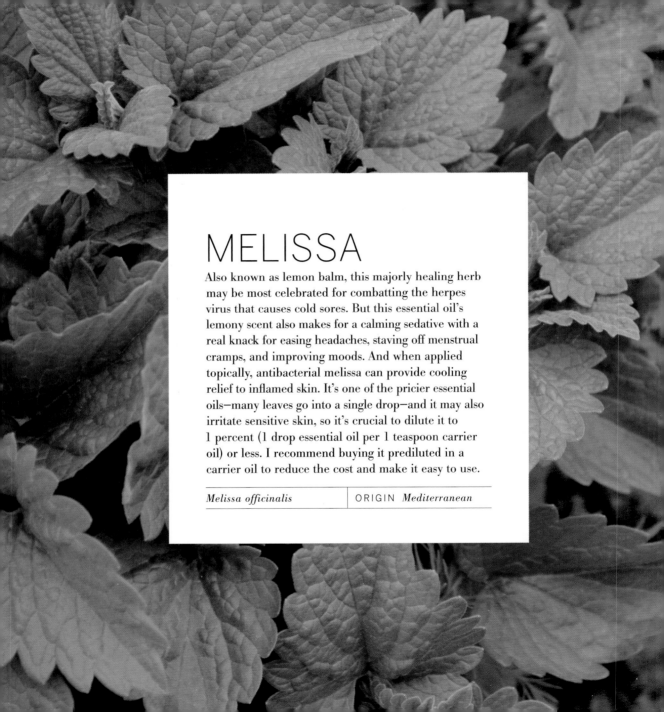

MELISSA

Also known as lemon balm, this majorly healing herb may be most celebrated for combatting the herpes virus that causes cold sores. But this essential oil's lemony scent also makes for a calming sedative with a real knack for easing headaches, staving off menstrual cramps, and improving moods. And when applied topically, antibacterial melissa can provide cooling relief to inflamed skin. It's one of the pricier essential oils—many leaves go into a single drop—and it may also irritate sensitive skin, so it's crucial to dilute it to 1 percent (1 drop essential oil per 1 teaspoon carrier oil) or less. I recommend buying it prediluted in a carrier oil to reduce the cost and make it easy to use.

| *Melissa officinalis* | ORIGIN *Mediterranean* |

Cold Sore Secret Weapon

3 tablespoons melissa-infused oil (see page 16)

1 tablespoon castor oil

1 tablespoon beeswax pellets

1 tablespoon mango butter

6 drops melissa essential oil

6 drops tea tree essential oil

10 drops lavender essential oil

3-ounce (90-mL) glass jar

The familiar tingle signaling that a cold sore is on the way always comes at the worst time. But you can keep cold sores in check by reducing stress (a common trigger) and speed up the healing process with this ointment, thanks to its anti-viral essential oils like melissa and tea tree, plus numbing peppermint for relief.

STEP 1 / Follow the directions on page 16 to make melissa-infused oil.

STEP 2 / Bring 2 inches (5 cm) of water to a boil in a small saucepan.

STEP 3 / Mix the melissa-infused oil, castor oil, beeswax, and mango butter in a heat-safe glass bowl. (Castor oil makes a great addition to lip balm recipes—it ups the gloss factor.)

STEP 4 / Turn the heat to low and place the bowl over the saucepan.

Heat until the ingredients have melted, stirring occasionally.

STEP 5 / Remove the oil mixture from the heat, and let it cool for 1 minute. Then stir in the melissa, tea tree, and lavender essential oils.

STEP 6 / Pour the mixture into your jar (or several smaller lip balm tins). Let it sit at room temperature until completely solid. Add the lid and store away from direct heat or sunlight; use within 8 months.

Spasm-Stopping Warm Compress

2 cups (475 mL) warm water

3 drops melissa essential oil

2 drops sweet marjoram essential oil

2 drops lavender essential oil

When a muscle cramp hits, a warm scented compress can help ease the ache and halt spasms by increasing blood flow to the area. Add soothing essential oils with pain-relieving and antispasmodic properties, such as melissa, which is especially helpful at relieving tummy cramps and backaches.

STEP 1 / Pour the warm water into a small bowl. Add the melissa, sweet marjoram, and lavender essential oils; stir well to disperse the oils.

STEP 2 / Soak a soft washcloth in the water. Squeeze out the excess water until it's wet but not dripping.

STEP 3 / Apply the cloth to the affected area. (It helps to hold a towel over the cloth to trap its heat.)

STEP 4 / Once the compress cools, repeat the process, continuing every 2 hours until no longer needed.

Cheerful Gel Air Fresheners

¾ cup (180 mL) water

¼-ounce (7-g) packet gelatin

8-ounce (240-mL) jar

¼ cup (60 mL) vodka

3 drops melissa essential oil

6 drops rose absolute
essential oil

4 drops lavender essential oil

1 to 2 drops natural food
coloring

Wick (optional)

Meet the gel air freshener—a superfun, strangely easy, and absolutely natural way to make your house smell great. You can customize this simple diffuser with your favorite scent, dye it a pretty pick-me-up color, and even add in fun decorative items, like shells or flowers. Then set it somewhere your house and enjoy! (You can even pop one in the fridge to combat food odors.) Go easy with the food coloring—you'll only need 1 to 2 drops for bright color.

STEP 1 / Bring the water to boil in a small saucepan. Add the gelatin packet and stir until it's completely dissolved. Remove from the heat and let sit until it's room temperature.

STEP 2 / Pour the gelatin-water mixture into your chosen jar, then add the vodka and the melissa, rose absolute, and lavender essential oils.

STEP 3 / To color your gel, experiment to find the hue you like best. To create soft tones, try diluting 1 drop natural food coloring in 1 cup (240 mL) water, then add drops of the diluted color to the mixture until you reach your desired hue.

STEP 4 / Gently stir in the food coloring (careful not to splash!) and then refrigerate until set.

STEP 5 / Place the air freshener around your house, wherever you can stop for a second and inhale the soothing scents. You can add a few more drops of essential oil on top to freshen it up as the days pass—it'll last up to 3 weeks.

TIP / You can also make a gel candle by attaching a wick to the bottom of your jar before adding the gelatin. Light the candle and the scent will get even more intense.

MORE GEL AIR FRESHENER IDEAS

Once you start crafting these neat diffusers, you won't want to stop! Try these combinations next.
PMS 4 drops each jasmine and geranium and 2 drops lemon.
CREATIVITY 7 drops lemon and 4 drops ylang ylang.

CLEANSING 2 drops lemongrass, 2 drops peppermint, and 9 drops palmarosa.
BURNOUT 6 drops sweet orange, 4 drops rosemary, and 3 drops geranium.

CLARITY 6 drops grapefruit, 4 drops pine, and 3 drops juniper berry.
COURAGE 5 drops rosemary, 7 drops cedarwood, and 1 drop vetiver.
GROUNDING 5 drops ginger and 4 drops each cardamom and black pepper.

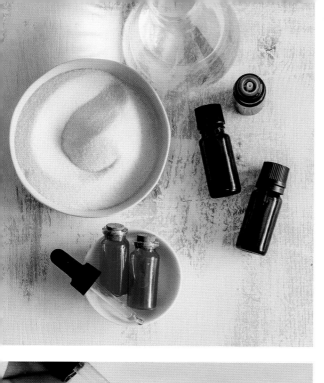

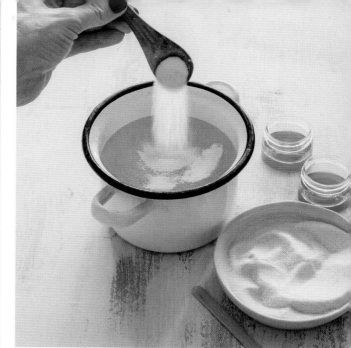

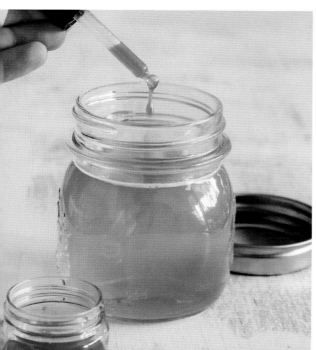

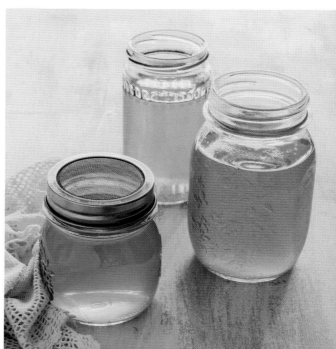

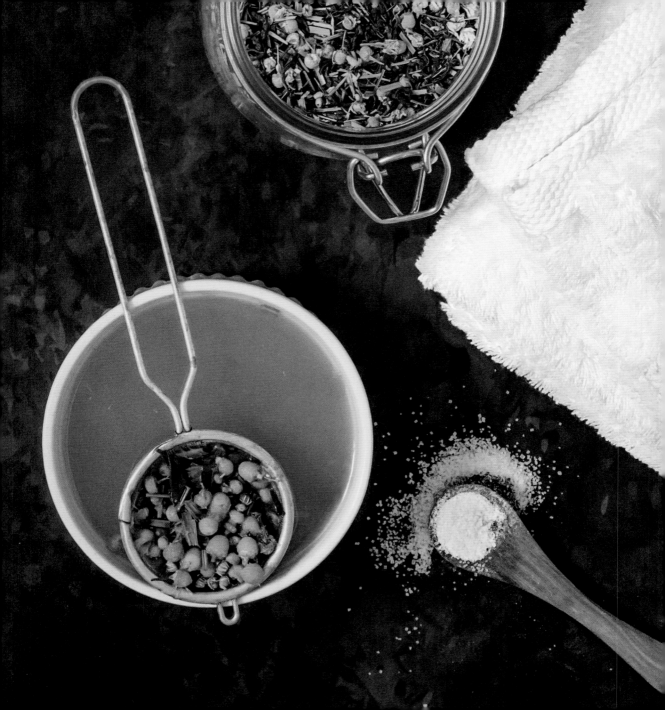

Recuperative Bath Infusion

2 cups (475 mL) water

1 tablespoon dried melissa

1 tablespoon dried chamomile

3 drops melissa essential oil

7 drops frankincense
essential oil

4 drops ylang ylang
essential oil

1 tablespoon sea salt

Who doesn't love seasonal summer herbs? But they're not just for the kitchen—they also make a wonderful addition to your beauty and wellness routines. Refresh your skin and spirits with this calming herbal bath "tea" infused with melissa and chamomile; it'll help alleviate anxiety, irritability, and insomnia.

STEP 1 / Bring the water to a boil. Pour it into a bowl containing the dried melissa and chamomile.

STEP 2 / Steep the mixture for 20 minutes, then strain out the herbs. (You can toss them right in the tub with you, but some—such as chamomile—break down in water and can be a pain to clean up.)

STEP 3 / In a separate bowl, drizzle the melissa, frankincense, and ylang ylang essential oils into the sea salt and stir together. Add the salt to the tea infusion and stir until dissolved.

STEP 4 / Pour the tea into a warm bath and enjoy your soak for 30 minutes—it'll help calm skin irritation and inflammation.

Skin-Rejuvenating Body Spray

1 cup (240 mL) water

1 green tea bag

½ cucumber

8-ounce (240-mL) spray bottle

2 tablespoons aloe vera gel

4 drops melissa essential oil

8 drops peppermint essential oil

Chilled green tea and cucumber sounds like the making of a heavenly poolside drink. And, in a way, it is—but for your skin. With this spray, harness green tea's anti-aging powers, plus the hydrating, skin-soothing benefits of cucumber and aloe vera and melissa's anti-inflammatory gifts. Little paper umbrella optional!

STEP 1 / Bring the water to a boil. Pour it over the green tea bag and steep for 5 minutes. Remove the bag and let the tea cool in the refrigerator.

STEP 2 / Peel and roughly chop half of a cucumber and puree it in a food processor or blender. (You should end up with about 6 tablespoons of juice.)

STEP 3 / Strain the pureed cucumber using a cheesecloth or a fine-mesh strainer; discard the solids.

STEP 4 / Add ½ cup (120 mL) tea to your spray bottle. (If your spray bottle is bigger, you can add more tea.)

STEP 5 / Add the strained cucumber juice, the aloe vera gel, and the melissa and peppermint essential oils to the spray bottle.

STEP 6 / Add the bottle's top and gently shake to combine. Spray generously, as it only lasts in the refrigerator for up to 2 weeks.

Common Ailments

Use this guide to discover the best oils for whatever you're fighting.
Remember to use them as topical treatments or inhalations—never ingest!

ACNE
Atlas cedarwood
Bergamot
Cypress
Geranium
Grapefruit
Lavender
Lemon
Oregano
Palmarosa
Rose
Rose geranium
Sandalwood
Sweet basil
Tea tree
Ylang ylang

ALLERGIES
Lavender
Lemon
Peppermint

ANGER
Bergamot
Lavender
Myrrh
Roman chamomile
Sweet orange
Vetiver
Ylang ylang

ANXIETY
Anise
Bergamot
Clary sage
Frankincense
Lavender
Roman chamomile

Rose
Sandalwood
Vetiver
Ylang Ylang

ARTHRITIS
Allspice
Birch
Black pepper
Carrot-seed
Cypress
Eucalyptus
Fennel
Juniper berry
Sweet basil

ATHLETE'S FOOT
Clove bud
Lavender
Lemon
Myrrh
Oregano
Palmarosa
Patchouli
Tea tree

BACK PAIN
Ginger
Juniper berry
Peppermint
Rosemary

BAD BREATH
Bergamot
Clove bud
Lavender
Peppermint

BLACKHEADS
Bergamot
Clary sage
Cypress
Eucalyptus
Lavender
Lemongrass
Thyme

BLISTERS
Lavender
Myrrh
Roman chamomile
Tea tree

BRUISES
Frankincense
Geranium
Helichrysum
Lavender

BUGS
Atlas cedarwood
Cajeput
Catnip
Citronella
Clove bud
Eucalyptus
Geranium
Lavender
Lemongrass
Oregano
Peppermint
Rose geranium
Rosemary
Tea Tree
Thyme

BUG BITES
Eucalyptus
Lavender
Roman chamomile
Rosemary
Sweet basil
Tea tree

BURNS
Carrot-seed
Geranium
German chamomile
Lavender
Roman chamomile
Tea tree

CELLULITE
Birch
Geranium
Grapefruit
Juniper berry
Lemon
Lemongrass
Lime
Patchouli
Pine
Rose geranium
Rosemary

CHAPPED LIPS
Geranium
Neroli
Roman chamomile
Rose geranium

COLDS
Benzoin
Black pepper

Camphor
Cinnamon bark
Eucalyptus
Ginger
Lavender
Lemon
Niaouli
Peppermint
Pine
Sweet basil
Tea tree
Thyme

COLD SORES
Bergamot
Lime
Melissa
Peppermint
Tea tree

CONGESTION
Eucalyptus
Oregano
Peppermint
Rosemary

COUGH
Allspice
Anise
Cardamom
Cinnamon bark
Cypress
Elemi
Eucalyptus
Lavender
Lemon
Oregano
Peppermint
Sweet basil

DANDRUFF
Atlas cedarwood
Bay
Lavender
Lemongrass
Manuka
Patchouli
Sandalwood
Tea tree
Ylang ylang

DEPRESSION
Allspice
Benzoin
Bergamot
Cassia bark
Cinnamon bark
Clary sage
Geranium
Ginger
Grapefruit
Jasmine
Lavender
Lemon verbena
Lime
Melissa
Neroli
Patchouli
Peppermint
Rose
Rose geranium
Rosemary

ECZEMA
Atlas cedarwood
Bay
Bergamot
Benzoin
Birch
Carrot-seed
Frankincense
Geranium
German chamomile
Helichrysum
Hyssop
Juniper berry
Lavender
Myrrh
Patchouli
Roman chamomile
Rose
Rose geranium
Sandalwood
Thyme
Vetiver

FATIGUE
Allspice
Black pepper
Carrot-seed
Citronella
Coriander
Frankincense
Grapefruit
Hyssop
Jasmine
Juniper berry
Lime
Palmarosa
Peppermint
Pine
Sweet basil
Ylang ylang

FOOT ODOR
Citronella
Cypress
Peppermint
Tea tree

FUNGAL INFECTIONS
Bay
Caraway seed
Cardamom
Cinnamon leaf
Clove bud
Coriander
Fennel
Fragonia
Ho wood
Kanuka
Lemon eucalyptus
Lemongrass
Manuka
May chang
Melissa
Niaouli
Oregano
Palmarosa
Patchouli
Peppermint
Rosalina
Rosewood
Spike lavender
Sweet marjoram
Tea tree
Thyme
Winter savory

GRIEF
Cypress
Frankincense
Helichrysum
Neroli
Rose
Sandalwood

HAIR LOSS
Bay
Melissa
Rosemary
Ylang ylang

HAY FEVER
Bergamot
Eucalyptus
Geranium
German chamomile
Lavender
Lemongrass
Melissa
Niaouli
Pine
Roman chamomile
Rose
Rose geranium
Rosemary
Rosewood
Tea tree
Ylang ylang

HEADACHES
Cajeput
Calamus
Cardamom
Cinnamon leaf
Citronella
German chamomile
Grapefruit
Lavender
Lemon
Lemongrass
Melissa
Neroli
Peppermint
Roman chamomile
Rose
Rosemary
Rosewood
Spearmint
Sweet basil
Sweet marjoram
Valerian

HIVES
German chamomile
Myrrh
Sweet basil

INGROWN HAIRS
Lavender
Roman chamomile
Tea tree

INSOMNIA
Clary sage
German chamomile
Juniper berry
Lavender
Mandarin
Neroli
Petitgrain
Roman chamomile
Rose
Spikenard
Vetiver

LEG CRAMPS
Geranium
Ginger
Hyssop
Helichrysum
Lavender
Rosemary
Sweet marjoram

MENOPAUSE
Atlas cedarwood
Bergamot
Black pepper
Cardamom
Cistus
Clary sage
Coriander
Cypress
Eucalyptus
Frankincense
Geranium
German chamomile
Ginger
Grapefruit
Helichrysum
Ho wood
Jasmine
Juniper berry
Lavender
Lemon
Lime
Mandarin
Neroli
Niaouli
Nutmeg
Palmarosa
Patchouli
Peppermint
Petitgrain
Plai
Roman chamomile
Rose
Rosemary
Sage
Sandalwood
Spearmint
Spikenard
Sweet basil

Sweet marjoram
Sweet orange
Thyme
Valerian
Vetiver
Vitex
Ylang ylang

MENSTRUAL CRAMPS
Anise
Black pepper
Cardamom
Clary sage
Cypress
Dill
Frankincense
Geranium
Ginger
Helichrysum
Juniper berry
Lavender
Melissa
Nutmeg
Peppermint
Plai
Roman chamomile
Rose
Sweet marjoram
Thyme

MOTION SICKNESS
Ginger
Grapefruit

NAIL CARE
Carrot-seed
Cypress
Frankincense
Grapefruit

Lavender
Lemon
Myrrh
Roman chamomile
Rosemary

NAIL FUNGUS
Clove bud
Lavender
Lemon
Oregano
Peppermint
Tea tree

NAUSEA
Allspice
Anise
Bergamot
Black pepper
Cardamom
Cassia bark
Coriander
Fennel
Geranium
German chamomile
Ginger
Grapefruit
Lavender
Lemongrass
Mandarin
Melissa
Peppermint
Roman chamomile
Rosewood
Spearmint
Spikenard
Sweet orange

OILY HAIR
Cypress
Eucalyptus
Lavender
Lemon
Rosemary
Sage
Sweet basil

PMS
Bergamot
Black pepper
Cardamom
Clary sage
Coriander
Cypress
Geramium
Grapefruit
Jasmine
Juniper berry
Lavender
Lemon
Niaouli
Nutmeg
Palmarosa
Peppermint
Petitgrain
Roman chamomile
Rose
Sweet basil
Sweet marjoram
Sweet orange
Vetiver
Ylang ylang

PSORIASIS
Atlas cedarwood
Bay
Bergamot

Birch
Cajeput
Clary sage
Geranium
German chamomile
Ho wood
Juniper berry
Lavender
Manuka
Roman chamomile
Rosewood
Sage
Spikenard
Tea tree

RAZOR BUMPS
Atlas cedarwood
Coriander
Eucalyptus
Geranium
German chamomile
Lavender
Manuka
Palmarosa
Peppermint
Roman chamomile
Sandalwood
Spearmint
Tea tree

ROSACEA
Bergamot FCF
  (furocoumarin-free)
Cypress
Eucalyptus
Frankincense
Geranium
German chamomile
Helichrysum

Ho wood
Juniper berry
Lavender
Manuka
Neroli
Oregano
Patchouli
Roman chamomile
Rose
Rosemary

SCARS
Benzoin
Elemi
Frankincense
Geranium
Helichrysum
Hyssop
Jasmine
Lavender
Mandarin
Manuka
Neroli
Palmarosa
Patchouli
Rose
Sandalwood
Tangerine

SORE/STIFF MUSCLES
Allspice
Anise
Benzoin
Birch
Black pepper
Calamus
Camphor
Carrot-seed
Clary sage

Clove bud
Coriander
Elemi
Eucalyptus
Fir needle
Ginger
Grapefruit
Jasmine
Juniper berry
Lavandin
Lavender
Lemongrass
Lime
Nutmeg
Palmarosa
Peppermint
Pine
Rosemary
Sage
Spearmint
Spruce
Sweet basil
Sweet marjoram
Thyme
Vetiver

STRESS
Allspice
Benzoin
Bergamot
Cardamom
Carrot-seed
Clary sage
Coriander
Cypress
Elemi
Geranium
German chamomile
Jasmine

Juniper berry
Lavandin
Lavender
Lemon
Lemon verbena
Lime
Mandarin
Melissa
Neroli
Palmarosa
Petitgrain
Pine
Roman chamomile
Rose
Rose geranium
Sandalwood
Spikenard
Spruce
Sweet marjoram
Sweet orange
Tangerine
Vanilla
Vetiver
Ylang ylang

STRETCH MARKS
Frankincense
Grapefruit
Helichrysum
Jasmine
Lavender
Mandarin
Manuka
Myrrh
Neroli
Roman chamomile
Rose
Sandalwood
Tangerine

SUNBURN
Eucalyptus
Geranium
German chamomile
Lavender
Peppermint
Tea tree

SWELLING
Cypress
Eucalyptus
Fennel
Grapefruit
Lavender
Lemongrass
Peppermint
Roman chamomile

VARICOSE VEINS
Cypress
Geranium
German chamomile
Juniper berry
Lavender
Lemon
Lemongrass
Lime
Niaouli
Peppermint
Roman chamomile
Rosemary
Spearmint
Spikenard

WARTS
Cinnamon leaf
Cypress
Geranium
Lavender
Lemon

Manuka
Neem
Niaouli
Oregano
Tea tree

WINTER BLUES
Bergamot
Clary sage
Cypress
Ginger
Grapefruit
Jasmine
Neroli
Sweet orange
Ylang ylang

WRINKLES
Carrot-seed
Frankincense
Geranium
Grapefruit
Lemon
Mandarin
Myrrh
Neroli
Roman chamomile
Rose
Rose geranium
Rosewood
Sandalwood
Tangerine
Vetiver
Ylang ylang

YEAST INFECTION
Myrrh
Oregano
Tea tree

Index

weldonowen

PRESIDENT & PUBLISHER
Roger Shaw
SVP, SALES & MARKETING
Amy Kaneko
SENIOR EDITOR Lucie Parker
EDITORIAL ASSISTANT
Molly O'Neil Stewart
CREATIVE DIRECTOR Kelly Booth
ART DIRECTOR Lorraine Rath
ASSOCIATE PRODUCTION DIRECTOR
Michelle Duggan
IMAGING MANAGER Don Hill

Weldon Owen is a division of
Bonnier Publishing USA.

1045 Sansome Street, Suite 100
San Francisco, CA 94111
www.weldonowen.com

Copyright © 2017 Weldon Owen Inc.

All rights reserved, including the
right of reproduction in whole or
in part in any form.

Library of Congress Cataloging in
Publication data is available.

ISBN: 1-978-168188-272-7

10 9 8 7 6 5 4 3 2 1
2017 2018 2019 2020 2021

Art Credits

ILLUSTRATION All illustrations by
Masako Kubo and Lorraine Rath.

PHOTOGRAPHY All photographs
by Ana Maria Stanciu unless
noted below.

Heidi's Bridge: 1, 59 Susan Hudson:
6, 118 Lindsey Johnson: 25, 73
bottom right, 74, 88, 93, 133, 152, 154
Stephanie Pollard: 16, 19, 37, 60, 67,
104, 109, 131, 140, 156 Shutterstock:
64, 98, 106, 114, 136, 155, 166, 172
Stocksy: 36, 82, 105, 144, 157

ART DIRECTION + DESIGN
Alisha Petro

Recipe Credits

Deborah Harju: 24 (all), 71 (bottom),
92 (top), 150 (all) Heidi's Bridge: 58
(top) Laura Heller: 71 (top) Lindsey
Johnson: 39, 69 (bottom), 121 (top),
143, 153 (top) Stephanie Pollard:
35 (top), 61, 66, 103 (bottom), 108,
130 (top), 139, 153 (bottom) Ashley
Poskin: 91, 149 Stephanie Stanesby:
26, 69 (top), 169

Author Acknowledgments

I've been so lucky to work with such
an amazing group of women to create
Hello Glow. Thank you to Stephanie
Pollard, Lindsey Johnson, and Deborah
Harju for creating so many smart,
beautiful, creative recipes—many that
you'll see in this book! And Ana Maria
Stanciu, I'm in serious awe of your
gorgeous photography. A big shout-
out to Kiersten Frase for keeping the
blog running while I worked on this
book. I can't even remember how I
managed without you!

Publisher Acknowledgments

Weldon Owen would like to thank Lisa
Marietta, Lily Miller, Marisa Solís, and
Kevin Broccoli and Laura Cheu of BIM
Creatives for editorial assistance.

Disclaimer

While every effort has been made
to provide accurate and up-to-date
information, the recipes, products,
and advice presented in this book
do not guarantee results and should
not be used for treating serious health
problems or diseases. Information
may change over time as further
research and clinical data become
available. If you have any concerns
about your skin, hair, or general health,
consult your personal healthcare
practitioner before applying any
recipe from this book. Always do
a patch test on a small area of the
skin, hair, fabric, floor, and any other
surfaces for any new products or
treatments. Use caution and monitor
flame when heating, melting, or
burning any of the ingredients
or products in this book to avoid
serious injury or fire. The author's
testimonials in this book represent
anecdotal experiences; individual
experiences will vary. Neither the
author nor the publisher may be held
responsible for claims resulting from
information in this book.

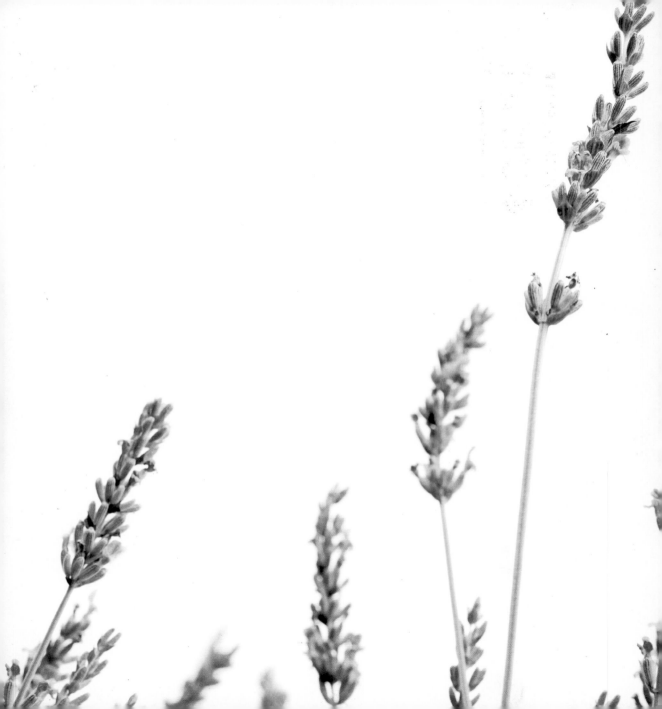